COMFORTING
the CONFUSED

2nd Edition

Stephanie B. Hoffman, PhD, is the Director of Interprofessional Team Training and Development and Primary Care Education at the James A. Haley Veterans' Hospital in Tampa, Florida. Dr. Hoffman is a life-span developmental psychologist. She has received funded grants to study the communication and management aspects of dementia, geriatric depression, feeding behavior in nursing-home residents, special care units, and restraint alternatives. At the James A. Haley Veterans' Hospital, Dr. Hoffman has trained hundreds of students and staff in the following disciplines: nursing, medicine, psychiatry, public health, medical records, pharmacy, podiatry, social work, speech pathology, audiology, occupational therapy, dietetics, physical therapy, and other associated health disciplines. Dr. Hoffman has conducted workshops on dementia management and team training throughout the country. She has published in the areas of geropsychology, dementia, team building, and nonverbal communication, and has written and edited several dementia-management books.

Constance A. Platt, MA, is a geropsychologist at the Binghamton Psychiatric Center in Binghamton, New York. Mrs. Platt conducts psychological assessments of psychiatric and dementia residents, practices individual and group psychotherapy, advises on the development of treatment plans, assists the interdisciplinary team on resident management issues, and has participated as a member of a geriatric mobile screening team. She teaches medical and psychology students and conducts nursing home inservice training sessions on dementia management and other long-term-care issues. Mrs. Platt serves as a consultant to nursing homes on the management of problem behaviors. She has received funded grants to study nonverbal communication and dementia and the impact of staff training on resident management, and she has published in these areas.

COMFORTING
the CONFUSED

2nd Edition

Strategies for
Managing Dementia

Stephanie B. Hoffman
Constance A. Platt

 Springer Publishing Company

Springer Publishing Company, Inc.
536 Broadway
New York, NY 10012-3955

Acquisitions Editor: Helvi Gold
Production Editor: Pamela Lankas
Cover design by James Scotto-Lavino

00 01 02 03 04 / 5 4 3 2 1

Library of Congress Cataloging-in-Publication Data

Hoffman, Stephanie B.
    Comforting the confused: strategies for managing dementia / Stephanie B. Hoffman and Constance A. Platt—2nd ed.
        p.   cm.
    Includes bibliographical references and index.
    ISBN 0-8261-1261-7 (softcover)
    1. Dementia.   2. Dementia—Patients—Care.   3. Interpersonal relations.   I. Platt, Constance A.   II. Title.
    [DNLM: 1. Dementia—psychology—Interpersonal Relations.
    2. Communication Disorders—psychology—Interpersonal Relations.
    WM 220 H711c 2000]
    RC521.H64 2000
    616.8'3—dc21   99-051495
                                                                CIP

Printed in the United States of America

Contents

Foreword

Confusion is a common symptom of brain dysfunction and occurs in a large percentage of elderly individuals. Several diseases may cause confusion, but the most common cause of confusion is Alzheimer's disease, either alone or in combination with cerebrovascular changes or with accumulation of Lewy bodies. Although major advances were made recently in investigating the causes of Alzheimer's disease and in developing new treatment strategies, we still do not have an effective cure for the disease, and it is unlikely that this cure will be discovered in the near future. Because the incidence of Alzheimer's disease increases with age and the number of aged individuals in our society is rapidly increasing, our society is faced with the challenge of caring for an increasing number of confused individuals.

Confusion is extremely stressful for the confused individual and complicates all personal interactions including provision of necessary care. Because we do not have an effective cure that will eliminate the confusion caused by Alzheimer's disease or most other brain dysfunction, comforting the confused is a major goal of care. Providing comfort may improve the quality of life of the confused individual even though it does not affect the underlying condition. Therefore, this book is extremely important because it describes strategies that comfort a demented individual.

An inability to communicate effectively is one of the main causes of confusion, and the authors appropriately start by describing the effects of aging and dementia on the ability to communicate and by explaining strategies that can maximize the ability to improve communication. However, comfort also may be diminished for other reasons, and the book discusses the issues of depression and behavioral symptoms of dementia, which can be both the cause and consequence of decreased comfort in a demented individual.

Assuring comfort in a confused individual is not an easy task. The concept of comfort includes not only a relief from discomfort, but also a state of ease, contentment, and transcendence (the ability to rise above problems or pain) (Kolcaba, 1991). Each of these three components of comfort occurs in four contexts: physical (bodily sensations), social (interpersonal and societal relationships), psychospiritual (internal awareness of self including esteem, sexuality, and meaning of one's life, as well as a relationship to a higher order or being), and environmental (light, noise, ambience, color, temperature, and esthetic values).

The degree of comfort perceived in a specific situation is highly individual and caregivers have to depend on subjective reports of care recipients in order to individualize care and maximize comfort. Such a report is difficult to obtain from a confused individual, who also may have speech impairment. The caregivers have to rely on careful assessment of both the physical and psychological state of the confused individual and on nonverbal communication. In general, it is easier to describe and measure discomfort than to define a comfort level (Hurley, Volicer, Hanrahan, Houde, & Volicer, 1992).

Comfort is important not only for demented individuals but also for their family members. Again, communication plays an important part in assuring comfort by providing agreement between family members and the staff regarding goals of care. Comfort may be the primary goal of care in managing individuals with advanced dementia. In this population, aggressive medical interventions produce a high degree of discomfort because the individuals do not understand the need for various treatments. Because the treatments also have a limited effectiveness, comfort may become more important than prolongation of life at all costs (Volicer & Hurley, 1998).

The usefulness of this book is enhanced by providing lists of learning objectives, and pretest and posttest questions for each chapter. The authors should be congratulated in providing a valuable tool for educating primary caregivers who care for confused individuals. I am sure that this book will provide significant contributions to our efforts to improve care for this vulnerable population.

LADISLAV VOLICER, MD, PHD
PROFESSOR OF PHARMACOLOGY AND PSYCHIATRY
BOSTON UNIVERSITY SCHOOL OF MEDICINE
CLINICAL DIRECTOR, GRECC

REFERENCES

Hurley, A. C., Volicer, B. J., Hanrahan, P., H ide, S., & Volicer, L. (1992). Assessment of discomfort in advanced Alzh mer patients. *Research in Nursing & Health, 15,* 369–377.

Kolcaba, K. Y. (1991). A taxonomic stru ire for the concept comfort. *IMAGE: Journal of Nursing Scholarship,* , 237–240.

Volicer, L., & Hurley, A. (1998). *Hospice ca for patients with advanced progressive dementia.* New York: Springer Pub hing Co.

Preface to the First Edition

A friendly face, a warm smile, a gentle touch, a soothing voice tone. All can improve the quality of life for those suffering from dementia.

Depression, withdrawal, rage, and poor communication are all symptoms of dementing illnesses. The dementia patient can feel intense frustration with memory losses and the inability to share, discuss, or confess fears about what is happening inside. The caregiver too is frustrated. But how to help? How to comfort? Research findings offer some ideas to caregivers and family members about how they can reach out to their relatives and patients (Hoffman, Platt, Barry, & Hamill, 1985).

Individuals with Alzheimer's disease and other brain disorders lose their ability to communicate verbally, both in terms of speaking to others and in understanding what is being said to them. We believe, however, that such persons retain an ability for communicating nonverbally—through touch, facial expression, voice tone, and body language. We suggest that the ability to communicate nonverbally may even sharpen as verbal abilities deteriorate, comparable to the more sensitive hearing of the blind.

To explore our idea, we conducted a study funded by the New York State Department of Health's Oxford Gerontology Center. We used actors to convey emotional messages to 10 cognitively intact residents and 40 residents with mild to severe cognitive impairment, all living in long-term-care facilities. Individuals were tested for their reactions to pleasant and unpleasant emotional messages presented through touch, voice tone, and facial expression. In the pleasant condition, the actor smiled at the resident, held a hand, and said the resident's name in a pleasant, soothing way. In the unpleasant condition, the actor frowned at the resident, clasped a wrist, and said the name sternly. Subjects were assessed for their reactions to the pleasant and unpleasant conditions. Videotapes of these interactions were rated for resident's eye contact, head and body orientation, and facial expression.

Results were very encouraging, showing that ability to respond to nonverbal messages is maintained, even in the profoundly demented. And even more important, demented individuals reacted positively to the pleasant approach and negatively to the unpleasant approach. In the positive condition, they smiled back at the actor, held onto the hand, and tried to maintain the interaction. In the negative condition, subjects were either startled or withdrew, frowning. This finding is extremely valuable, as it demonstrates that caregivers' emotions are transmitted nonverbally to demented residents. If a caregiver is warm and friendly, residents respond in a similar manner and thus will be much easier to handle. If a caregiver is upset or angry, the residents will similarly tend to respond in an upset or hostile way.

Caregivers of persons with dementia may not be aware of the way they and the residents communicate nonverbally. Based on our research findings, we believe that caregivers should be instructed and encouraged to emphasize nonverbal aspects of their communication when caring for the demented; a warm touch, a calming tone of voice, a friendly smile, all would do much to alleviate frustration and improve understanding between patient and caregiver. We wrote this book to provide both an understanding of why communication is so difficult with demented individuals and some strategies for managing their behavioral problems. As a result of applying these techniques, we believe that both the caregivers and residents will be comforted. The confusion of caregivers about how to handle demented individuals, in addition to demented individuals' confusion as a result of their disease, may be lessened.

Demented residents can be said to be confused, although confusion is a term that is not well understood. According to Wolanin and Phillips (1981), "the term *confusion,* while used freely by health professionals, is not clearly defined. It is a label for behaviors that caregivers recognize as being deviant from those expected from the client in a certain place and at a certain time." Confusion is a symptom with different meanings to different people, as we all have very different expectations about what is appropriate behavior. Anything that differs from appropriate behavior and feelings might be called confusion. We, as caregivers, can also be considered confused if our own feelings and behaviors are different from what we expect of ourselves. Caregivers might believe that they should be able to manage demented individuals calmly and professionally, yet in actuality find themselves burned out, frustrated, or unsure.

As your understanding of the behaviors of demented persons and their caregivers becomes clearer, you may have far different ideas at the book's conclusion about what are appropriate behaviors and emotions for both demented individuals and their caregivers. There may be far less confusion as all are comforted by increased caregiving knowledge and skills. This book is designed for personal reading and for classroom or in-service training. We encourage readers to analyze the objectives, take the pretests and posttests, and engage in the learning exercises at the end of each chapter. Most of the information is, of course, understood best through "hands-on" practice. Please try out our techniques, see through new eyes, and understand through new concepts. Others who have had our training have said they've been greatly helped by the material in these chapters.

REFERENCES

Hoffman, S. B., Platt, C. A., Barry, K. E., & Hamill, L. A. (1985). When language fails: Nonverbal communication abilities of the demented. In J. T. Hutton & A. D. Kennedy (Eds.), *Senile dementia of the Alzheimer type* (pp. 49–64). New York: Alan R. Liss.

Wolanin, M. O., & Philips, L. R. F. (1981). *Confusion: Prevention and care.* St. Louis: C. V. Mosby.

Preface to the Second Edition

In the 10 years since the publication of our first edition, the field of Alzheimer's disease has exploded. Hundreds of researchers all over the world are making significant strides in our understanding of the etiology and diagnosis of the disorder. Several promising drugs are on the horizon that will prevent or slow dementing changes to the brain. However, little in the way of new behavioral treatments has been discovered to deal with the frustrating and perplexing behavioral problems of persons with Alzheimer's disease (AD) and other dementing disorders. Our comforting strategies, proposed since the early 1990s, are still critically important in the management of those with AD. If anything, they are even more important, as a well-informed public grows increasingly anxious as they age and some begin to experience cognitive decline.

Thank you for using our new book and trying our approaches. We've updated our material to reflect scientific advances in our understanding of dementia. We've also included some important new chapters on special care units, feeding, restraints, and dying/grieving. If you study our strategies carefully, you will find yourself feeling much more comfortable in your vital role as caregiver to people with dementia.

Acknowledgments

We thank the New York State Department of Health and the Oxford Gerontology Center for their funding of the studies that prompted this book and the residents, families, and staff who participated in our research and training programs. A very special thank you to Kathleen Barry-Wacaser, who was the project assistant on two of our studies. Dr. Barry-Wacaser was instrumental in the development and evaluation of a training manual on dementia management. She showed unusual talent in the conduct of the research assessing the communication abilities of dementia residents and in training staff to use nonverbal communication techniques. We also thank Lynn Hamill Hughes who worked with us on our original research study and who contributed greatly to the success of our efforts.

We thank the Binghamton Psychiatric Center for their encouragement of our research efforts, and Rivermede Nursing Home for their participation in our training program evaluation. The Clinical Campus of Upstate Medical Center was exceptionally supportive of our research efforts, providing much in the way of administrative assistance and encouragement. The success of the research was in large part due to their help.

We would like to acknowledge Peggy Bargmann, RN, and Sue Miller, RN, C, MSN, of the Hillhaven Corporation, for their hospitality and comments concerning the Special Care Unit for dementia at the Carrollwood Care Center.

Thank you to our husbands, families, and colleagues for encouraging us during the preparation of this book.

We wish to thank the individuals with dementia whose cases we have cited to demonstrate a point in our text. Their names and identifying information have been changed to protect anonymity. Some cases are composites of several persons.

Introduction: Dementia—An Overview

LEARNING OBJECTIVES

- To recognize that disorientation, memory loss, and confusion result from many causes, some reversible and some irreversible.
- To identify common symptoms of dementia.
- To identify causes of stress in those providing care for demented residents.
- To develop an awareness of emotional responses to demented residents.

PRETEST

In the following spaces, place a "T" before true statements, an "F" before false statements, and a question mark before those you don't know.

_____ 1. Dementia is a recently discovered illness.

_____ 2. Dementia is always irreversible.

_____ 3. If you were to ask dementia residents to explain the proverb, "A stitch in time saves nine," they probably could.

_____ 4. Caring for individuals with dementia can be stressful to caregivers.

_____ 5. Depression often accompanies dementia.

_____ 6. Technologies that sharply image the brain are used to help diagnose dementia.

_____ 7. Of those over age 80, nearly 50% may have severe dementia.

_____ 8. Safety is usually not a problem for dementia residents.

_____ 9. Over time, individuals with dementia often forget who their close friends and family are.

_____ 10. Individuals with dementia gradually lose their ability to use language.

One of the greatest fears about getting old is becoming demented. The loss of mental or cognitive abilities is what is medically known as dementia. In recent years, there has been a dramatic amount of attention directed at studying dementing illnesses (Progress Report on Alzheimer's Disease, 1998). Many exciting breakthroughs have been made in defining the characteristics and causes of dementia. Most researchers now agree that dementia is a symptom of a disease process—that it is not a natural and normal part of aging (Katzman, 1986; Wurtman, 1985). The symptoms of dementia may be caused by more than 70 known diseases, but Alzheimer's disease alone accounts for more than half the cases (Katzman, Lakser, & Bernstein, 1988).

THE HISTORY OF DEMENTIA

Mahendra (1984) and Torack (1983) have written fascinating histories of the concept of dementia, tracing references to it from the time of Cicero in the second century B.C. through various philosophers, poets, and physicians, to the first scientific report of a specific brain disease by Alois Alzheimer in 1907. Cicero noted that the "senile folly called dotage" (Torack, 1983) was characteristic of only frivolous old men. And the famous Roman physician, Galen, discussed the disease called morosis, which affected knowledge and memory in some of the old people. Mahendra notes that the term "dementia" comes from the Latin word "dementatus," which means "out of one's mind, crazed, applicable to any and all abnormal, unusual, incomprehensible or bizarre behavior" (Mahendra, 1984). Mahendra comments that dementia was rare in early cultures as few people lived to old age. For many centuries, dementia and old age were thought to necessarily occur together. Even Shakespeare in his play *As You Like It* refers to old age as a second childishness without touch, eyes, taste, everything. British medical practitioners in the 1600s had such curious expressions for

---

Answers: 1-F, 2-F, 3-F, 4-T, 5-T, 6-F, 7-T, 8-F, 9-T, 10-T.

dementia as "fatuitas or stultitia," and described a man as "decayed in his intellectuals." The mental changes caused by syphilis, some say introduced to Europe by Christopher Columbus after his return from Haiti in 1493, complicated the diagnostic picture for decades. Mahendra discusses the idea that witches, persecuted in the 17th and 18th centuries, may have been suffering from dementia. In the 1800s the classification of dementia made a major leap forward with various physicians, such as Cullen, Rush, Pinel, and Esquirol, distinguishing it from mental retardation and syphilitic paresis and attributing it to other disease states, such as that of the cerebral arteries. Brain diseases discovered by Huntington, Pick, Binswanger, and Kraepelin were described in that century as well. But it was Alzheimer in the early twentieth century who observed the clinical presentation of a brain illness—"morbid jealousy, loss of memory, capricious behavior, spatial and temporal disturbances, persecutory ideas, and speech difficulties" (Mahendra, 1984)—in a 51-year-old woman and the microscopic brain changes of plaques and tangles characteristic of Alzheimer's disease.

SYMPTOMS OF DEMENTIA

Mrs. Forrest, 64 years old, often forgets where she leaves her car keys. She has been sleeping badly. Her performance at work was recently rated as poor because of increasing confusion and inability to follow directions. She cannot recall anyone's name anymore, even close friends and family.

Howard Stevens, 77 years old, was taken by his wife and son to the Memory Disorders Clinic for a complete evaluation. During the past 18 months, he began to forget the way home from the grocery store. He becomes very angry if you ask him a question he can't answer. And he always loses his train of thought in the middle of a sentence. Although Mr. Stevens seems to be working on the checkbook, many bills are now marked "past due." Sometimes he can't make it to the bathroom on time. However, he denies that anything is wrong with him—he says most of his friends are having similar problems.

Mrs. Kramer, who is 84, paces the building all day. She says she is looking for her sister's house and asks where it is. Mrs. Kramer is tearful, anxious, and confused, though her children report that she was always very poised and calm in the past. She thinks her roommate is trying to kill her and has been moved three times already. She constantly curses at the staff, though her family reports that she used to be a very gracious lady, who did not seem to ever use bad language.

What are the symptoms of dementing disorders? Memory loss, especially for recent events, is the most typical sign of dementia. It is also often the earliest sign of the disease. If a person is unable to remember a list of three objects after five minutes, she is considered to have impairment of recent memory (American Psychiatric Association, 1994). This is also demonstrated in everyday life by being unable to recall what was eaten for breakfast, or as dementia gets worse, that breakfast was even eaten at all. Long-term memory, the ability to remember events and things from the past, may also be impaired in dementia, especially in later stages of a progressive brain illness. A demented individual might not be able to remember his or her place and date of birth. A man may not remember that he was married, or that his current visitor is his wife of 50 years. Disorientation is a type of memory loss as well. Disorientation means that a person does not notice or remember the basic facts of existence—where the person is, who the person is, or what time it is.

Other symptoms, in addition to memory loss, are characteristic of dementia. Various aspects of cognitive functioning are affected by dementing illnesses. What is cognition? *Taber's Cyclopedic Medical Dictionary* (Thomas, 1981) defines cognition as "awareness with perception, reasoning, intuition, and memory; the process by which knowledge is acquired." All of these aspects of cognition and other brain functions can be affected by dementia. According to the American Psychiatric Association (1994), a person must show at least one of these other symptoms along with memory loss to be diagnosed as demented. This includes poor judgment, such as going out on a cold day without a warm coat or trying to cook food in a plastic dish on a gas stove. Another dementia symptom is impairment of abstract thinking. Demented persons interpret what you say very literally. They cannot understand proverbs such as "a rolling stone gathers no moss." A demented individual also cannot reason clearly. In early stages of the disease, the person may rely on problem-solving strategies that have always worked in the past, though now that conditions have changed, these are no longer effective. For instance, if there was trouble at work in the past, the person might have stayed later and worked longer hours to get the work done. With dementia, however, working longer hours will not help reasoning abilities. The person may be making very poor decisions. Many wives have reported that their husbands with dementia almost ruined the family business before the wives became aware of the extent of their husbands' problems.

Disturbances of other brain functions, such as the ability to use language, carry out motor tasks, follow complicated directions, manage money, recognize objects or people, or construct things, can be symptoms of dementia. Personality change, in terms of either a change in or an exaggeration of previous personality traits, is another symptom of dementia.

The above changes must be great enough to interfere with the person's ability to work or get along with other people. Also, the symptoms cannot be due to an acute physical problem that is affecting the brain (American Psychiatric Association, 1994). If, for example, the changes are acute rather than chronic and accompanied by fluctuations in consciousness, disturbed perceptions, and rich fantasies, the person is suffering from a delirium rather than a dementia (Jenike, 1989; Lipowski, 1983).

Language difficulties common in dementia affect the person's ability to name things or say what the person wants to say (Appell, Kertesz, & Fishman, 1982). This is in fact a very early indication of the disease. Other characteristics of demented persons include an appearance of frustration, withdrawal, suspiciousness, irritability, and restlessness. They may spend their days wandering around their residence. They may be disoriented and not know where they are or what time of day it is. Dementia residents have changes in their sleep cycle—they may be wakeful at night and take cat naps all day. They may lose the ability to care for their daily needs, forget how to dress, become incontinent, become unable to walk, or feed themselves. These motor changes, which occur late in the disease, can mean that a dementia resident will not be able to swallow or even figure out how to sit down in a chair.

Dementia residents often are no longer able to recognize close friends or family members, or even themselves. Demented individuals may become frightened at their own face in the mirror, thinking that a stranger is looking at them.

Catastrophic reactions may occur, such as bursts of anger or crying when unable to perform as before or when in a frustrating situation. Symptoms may get worse in the evening—this is known as "sundowning." Depression as a reaction to these changes is often present, especially in early stages of dementia (Aronson, Gaston, & Merriam, 1984; Katz, Aronson, & Lipkowitz, 1982). Not all individuals will become depressed. If they do experience depression, their depression will probably lift at moderate or later stages of their dementing illness. However, it is important for depression to be diagnosed and treated in all persons with dementia, as it will contribute to excess disability.

Demented persons will also be confused, although as noted in the preface, confusion is a term that is not well defined. However, they do tend to act in ways that are inappropriate to the time and place because of poor impulse control.

PERSONALITY CHANGES IN DEMENTIA

Damage to the brain often causes a release of inhibitions on behavior. The person is no longer as able to avoid acting on impulse and may engage in destructive, inappropriately sexual, verbally abusive or physically aggressive behavior. Parts of the brain responsible for control of such impulses are damaged and can no longer exercise control. The individual cannot avoid swearing, moaning, crying, hitting out, masturbating, or acting in very self-centered ways. Although as caregivers we may feel that dementia residents are doing things "on purpose," they may be unable to control their behavior and should not be blamed for it.

Also, persons with dementia are often aware of their inability to perform as they once did. This contributes to their own emotional reactions to their problems. Especially in the early stages of the disease, individuals may be aware of their mental failings and become depressed, withdrawn, enraged, or lash out. Feeling yourself change without any way to stop such changes can also cause tremendous anxiety. Demented individuals may cope with this anxiety in ways that have worked for them in the past, only more so. If the person drank alcohol to cope with anxiety, he may be drunk all the time. If your mother became demanding when she didn't feel good, she may become even more demanding and manipulative as a way to seek comfort. This can be very stressful to the caregiver. Also stressful are the paranoia and delusions or hallucinations that sometimes accompany dementia. If the person forgets where something is, the caregiver may be accused of stealing it, as it is easier to blame others than to blame oneself. Demented individuals may think that people are out to get them, may see visions or hear things that aren't there, or think that television characters are real people. They may become panicked when unable to recognize the caregiver. These are all very common changes, though that doesn't make them easier to deal with.

CAUSES OF DEMENTIA

Memory loss, disorientation, and confusion can have many causes. Also, more than one cause can be present in the person having these symptoms. For example, a resident may have recently relocated, be on several medications, have an acute urinary tract infection, be depressed, and have mild Alzheimer's disease. All these factors would contribute to confusion and memory loss. Some of the causes of dementia are reversible. That is, if the person showing these symptoms is diagnosed and receives treatment for the underlying condition causing the symptoms, mental functioning will improve. However, many of the causes of dementia are irreversible. They can not at this time be prevented or reversed, although the symptoms can be treated to make an individual more comfortable. The conditions labeled as irreversible causes of dementia are currently only irreversible because we have not yet discovered a cure for the disease. With time and further research, it is hoped that many of the conditions considered to cause irreversible dementia may soon become treatable (Katzman et al., 1988).

Reversible Dementias

Reversible dementias are associated with acute disease or trauma to the brain. Doctors often refer to reversible dementias as delirium or acute brain syndrome. Another type of reversible dementia is "pseudodementia" or the confusion and memory loss associated with depression. The person with pseudodementia or the dementia of depression is often disoriented and apathetic, answering "I don't know" to most questions and complaining of memory loss (Wells, 1979). As symptoms of depression often mimic symptoms of dementia, it is at times difficult to know if a person is showing signs of dementia due to depression or is depressed due to the experience of dementia. Treatment for depression improves memory function in the person with pseudodementia.

Irreversible Dementias

The irreversible dementias were in the past known as chronic brain syndrome. They involve changes in brain structure of a permanent nature. Nerve cells die and important brain chemicals that control communication between nerve cells are depleted. With some brain diseases, senile plaques, tangles, and deposits are present in specific areas of the brain. Diagnosis of an irreversible dementia necessitates medical tests to rule out other more acute conditions. These tests can include the CT scan, MRI, EEG, blood analysis, mental status and neurological exams, and review of medications (Katzman et al., 1988). If these tests show that the memory impaired or disoriented person has no underlying acute problem, an irreversible dementia is suspected. However, a definitive diagnosis of Alzheimer's disease is usually not possible until an autopsy of the brain is performed.

TYPES OF BRAIN DISORDERS

Alzheimer's disease and multiinfarct dementia are the two major irreversible brain illnesses. Each of these dementias will be discussed in depth in following chapters. Dementias associated with multiple sclerosis and AIDS will also be discussed in the chapter dealing with younger patients. Other less common dementing illnesses include frontal lobe dementia, Pick's disease, Lewy body dementia, Huntington's disease, Cruetzfeldt-Jakob disease, Wernicke-Korsakoff syndrome, neurosyphilis, and the dementia associated with Parkinson's disease (Bayles & Kaszniak, 1987; Davis & Robertson, 1997; McKeith et al., 1996; U.S. Congress, 1987).

Frontal lobe dementia is characterized by changes in personality, motivation, social interaction, and organizational abilities (Gregory & Hodges, 1996). Speech is also affected, eventually resulting in the person becoming completely mute (Talbot, 1996). Persons with this disease may develop a "sweet tooth" and other compulsions (Miller et al., 1995).

Pick's disease is very similar to Alzheimer's disease, except that it has an earlier onset, usually in the mid-50's. The brains of these patients have plaques and tangles plus Pick cells, which look like neurons swollen into a balloon shape. Most of the brain cell damage is in the frontal lobe, so patients have profound personality change as the first symptom of the disease. They will demonstrate emotional lability, disinhibition, lack of insight, and lack of social awareness.

Lewy body dementia is a syndrome presenting mainly with visual hallucinations, delusions, as well as other cognitive problems. There are also periods of delirium and mild Parkinson-like symptoms. Persons with Lewy body disease have many side effects to neuroleptic medications (Burke, Pfeiffer, & McComb, 1998).

Huntington's disease, also known as Huntington's chorea, has a middle-aged age of onset, usually between ages 35 to 50. This is a hereditary, progressive disease that affects both cognitive and physical functioning as well as personality. The chorea involves jerky movements which cannot be controlled by the individual. Face, neck, and arms are affected early, as well as speaking ability. This disease is inherited from a parent with the illness, with the child having a 50 percent chance of inheriting it.

Cruetzfeldt-Jakob disease has a typical onset in middle age. This rare disease has an extremely rapid onset. The disease is caused by a slow virus. Symptoms of the illness include rapid changes in vision or hearing, a decrease in muscle strength, difficulty with coordination, and sudden dementia.

Wernicke-Korsakoff syndrome is a brain illness usually brought on by chronic alcohol intake. It is related to poor nutrition, especially an inadequate amount of thiamin. If the disease is treated quickly enough with nutritional supplements, the early Wernicke's confusion may be reversible. Korsakoff's is especially characterized by loss of recent memory and disorientation to time.

Neurosyphilis is increasingly rare, as syphilis is now easily treated. However, some older adults may not have been diagnosed or adequately treated for the illness. They will show a dementia anywhere from two to thirty years after infection.

Parkinson's disease itself may cause a difficulty in reasoning and the ability to handle unusual situations—the person may cope well in everyday routine, but will have difficulty adjusting to new problems (Boller, 1985; Taylor, Saint-Cyr, & Lang, 1986). The individual may also have problems with directions, with balance, and with constructing objects. Parkinson's disease causes resting tremor, rigidity, slowness, stooped posture, difficulty in starting to move, a freezing of movement, a flat facial expression, and in some persons a difficulty in speaking and writing (Glickstein, 1988). The severity of symptoms increases over time. These problems are due to the loss of cells in the substantia nigra of the brain, which produce dopamine. Patients with Parkinson's disease can get some relief from levodopa treatment during the middle stage of the disease.

Normal pressure hydrocephalus, a somewhat rare problem, causes a dementia that is actually reversible in some individuals if it is treated. Normal pressure hydrocephalus stems from pressure on the brain as fluid builds up in the ventricles. Its three main characteristics are a wide-based gait, urinary incontinence, and dementia. If a shunt is inserted, which drains the fluid from the ventricles, dementia may lessen.

RISK OF DEVELOPING DEMENTIA

Although the prevalence of dementia is quite low in the young-old (those aged 65–74), it is true that the risk of developing a dementing illness increases steadily with advancing age, such that almost 50% of those 85 and older will have a dementing illness (Hendrie, 1998). Younger persons are at much less risk of developing a dementia, unless they contract multiple sclerosis, Huntington's disease, brain infections, AIDS, or suffer brain injury in some way. However, there is a familial form of Alzheimer's disease that does affect a very small percentage of people younger than age 65. This is a more severe form of the disease, and it does have a higher likelihood of being genetically inherited (Heston, 1985).

CARING FOR THE DEMENTIA RESIDENT

Caring for the demented person can be a great source of stress to the caregiver (Cantor, 1983; Mace & Rabins, 1981). Why is it so difficult? One area that causes difficulty is the tremendous responsibility that comes with caring for someone who has poor judgment. The caregiver is responsible for the demented person's health and safety, and the resident may be behaving in very unhealthy and unsafe ways. For instance, residents may be so restless that they walk up and down a corridor all day to the point of exhaustion. They may wander outside, risking getting lost or hit by a car. They may put things in their mouth, risking germs, poisoning, and choking. They may also have developed distorted sleep patterns so that they are awake at night disturbing others. These behaviors are very difficult for many caregivers to manage, often because of the worry that if the demented person is not watched every minute, some harm will befall the individual.

Caregivers may also have concerns for their own personal safety. Dementia residents often have periods of being aggressive and unpredictable. Because of poor memory, poor judgment, and loss of impulse control, they may strike out at even the most sympathetic caregiver. Although the person is not behaving this way on purpose, caregivers may feel upset that their efforts are not being appreciated, and there may be concern about personal physical safety. Violent episodes are rare and can usually be controlled with a calm, positive approach or medications.

Social support issues also make caring for a dementia resident stressful. Caregivers may view caring for dementia residents as a low status, thankless task to be avoided if possible. Or they may not understand why it should be so difficult. The family of the dementia resident may be overly critical of staff's efforts, which can be a reaction to their own feelings of guilt over not caring for their relative themselves. The residents themselves may be unable to show affection or appreciation to the caregiver. A caregiver may then be constantly on the giving end.

Communication difficulties with the dementia resident are also stressful. People who first spoke another language will revert to that language, making communication difficult with English-speaking caregivers. Persons with Alzheimer's disease typically become progressively more disabled in their language ability to the point where they may have no useful speech at all. And understanding of the words of others becomes equally impaired, though demented persons are still responsive to nonverbal cues. They also often show a delayed reaction time, so that even when they can answer a question, it takes a very long time for them to respond. Their memories are so poor that they ask you the same question over and over again, forgetting the answer immediately. These problems make communication with the dementia resident very frustrating and time-consuming.

Emotional Reactions

What emotional reactions do caregivers experience in working with demented individuals? One common reaction is fear for the future—"I may get like that some day." Other reactions can include pity, guilt, irritation, helplessness, depression, anger. Feelings of stress and burnout are common. But these are all negative emotional reactions. Caring for dementia residents can lead to positive feelings as well. Caregivers can get very attached to those in their care. Their obvious dependency can lead caregivers to feelings of protectiveness, responsibility, and wanting to nurture. The rewards can be a smile, a hand clasp, or just knowing they are really needed.

SUMMARY

An overview of dementia is presented, with characteristic symptoms and diseases reviewed and caregiver stresses outlined. This introduction touches on material that will be covered in more depth in future chapters of this book: sensory changes, communication strategies, Alzheimer's disease, vascular dementia, depression, problem-solving strategies for caregivers, wandering, feeding problems, caring for younger residents, and family issues.

LEARNING EXERCISES

1. What does it feel like to be disoriented?

   • Think of a personal example of disorientation, e.g. waking up in a strange place, losing your car in a mall parking lot, or the effects of surgical anesthesia on your sense of time.
   • List the feelings these experiences aroused in you.
   • Discuss how feelings of disorientation may affect demented residents.

2. If you are currently a caregiver, what are your sources of stress in caring for dementia residents? List all the stressful situations and problems that confront you personally in providing care to someone who is demented.

3. If you are a caregiver, what are your emotional reactions to caring for dementia residents? List all your emotions which occur either in providing care or in observing changes in the resident.

4. Case Study of Joe

> *Joe, 84, spends his day wandering in the hall, tinkering with doorknobs, handrails, anything mechanical, and mumbling to himself. Often, toward evening, he will quite anxiously stop you and ask you to give him a ride, as he has to get home to help his mother milk the cows. He doesn't seem to understand your explanation that he is in a nursing home now and keeps repeating his need to get home to milk the cows. Sometimes when you try to take Joe to his room to prepare him for bed, he will pull away from you roughly and keep walking. Once you got hurt by him in this way, but you don't feel he intentionally hurt you. Even though you've worked with Joe for over a year, he doesn't know your name although he seems to recognize you at times. Sometimes he gives you a big smile and calls you "Fran." You wonder who Fran is and what is going on in his mind.*
>
> *Joe needs help dressing now, and he's losing weight too, so his clothes don't fit well. He's having trouble at mealtimes. He seems to forget why he's there and needs to be reminded to finish eating—and sometimes he'll use his hands instead of his fork and spoon, coughing throughout the meal.*
>
> *His daughter visits him once a month, but Joe doesn't seem to remember when she's been there. She doesn't stay long because he doesn't recognize her and can't carry on much of a conversation.*

*   What symptoms of dementia is Joe exhibiting?
*   What concerns would you have in caring for someone like Joe?

POSTTEST

Place a "T" before true statements, an "F" before false statements, and a question mark before those you don't know.

_____ 1. Dementia is the medical term for loss of cognitive abilities.

_____ 2. Dementia is a natural result of old age.

_____ 3. Individuals with dementia sometimes have poor impulse control.

_____ 4. Dementia impairs short-term memory.

_____ 5. Someone can appear to have dementia but really be very depressed instead.

_____ 6. Irreversible dementia results from the death of nerve cells in the brain.

_____ 7. An accurate diagnosis of dementia can be made on the basis of CT scan alone.

_____ 8. Dementia can occur with or without depression.

_____ 9. Alzheimer's disease is the most common kind of irreversible dementia.

_____ 10. An individual with dementia can think and reason clearly— only memory is affected.

REFERENCES

American Psychiatric Association. (1994). *Diagnostic and statistical manual of mental disorders (4th ed.)*. Washington, DC: American Psychiatric Press.

Appell, J., Kertesz, A., & Fishman, M. (1982). A study of language functioning in Alzheimer's patients. *Brain and Language, 17,* 73–91.

Aronson, M., Gaston, F., & Merriam, A. (1984). Depression associated with dementia. *Generations, 9,* 49–51.

Bayles, K. A., & Kaszniak, A. W. (1987). *Communication and cognition in normal aging and dementia.* Boston: Little, Brown.

Boller, F. (1985). Parkinson's disease and Alzheimer's disease: Are they associated? In J. T. Hutton & A. D. Kenney (Eds.), *Senile dementia of the Alzheimer type* (pp. 119–129). New York: Alan R. Liss.

Burke, W. J., Pfeiffer, R. F., & McComb, R. D. (1998). Neuroleptic sensitivity to closapine in dementia with Lewy bodies. *Journal of Neuropsychiatry & Clinical Neurosciences, 10,* 227–229.

Cantor, M. H. (1983). Strain among caregivers. *Gerontologist, 26,* 597–604.

Davis, R. L., & Robertson, E. M. (1997). *Textbook of neuropathology* (3rd ed.). Baltimore: Williams & Wilkins.

Glickstein, J. K. (1988). Managing the client with Parkinson's disease. *Focus on Geriatric Care and Rehabilitation, 2*(6), 2–3.

Gregory, C. A., & Hodges, J. R. (1996). Clinical features of frontal lobe dementia in comparison to Alzheimer's disease. *Journal of Neural Transmission. Supplementum, 47,* 103–123.

Answers: 1-T, 2-F, 3-T, 4-T, 5-T, 6-T, 7-F, 8-T, 9-T, 10-F.

Hendrie, H. C. (1998). Epidemiology of dementia and Alzheimer's disease. *American Journal of Geriatric Psychiatry, 6*(2) S3–S18.

Heston, L. (1985). Clinical genetics of Alzheimer's disease. In J. T. Hutton & A. D. Kenney (Eds.), *Senile dementia of the Alzheimer type* (pp. 197–204). New York: Alan R. Liss.

Jenike, M. A. (1989). *Geriatric psychiatry and psychopharmacology.* Chicago: Year Book Medical Publishers.

Katz, I., Aronson, M., & Lipkowitz, R. (1982). Depression secondary to dementia presents an ongoing dilemma. *Generations,* pp. 24–25.

Katzman, R. (1986). Alzheimer's disease. *New England Journal of Medicine, 314,* 964–973.

Katzman, R., Lasker, B., & Bernstein, N. (1988). Advances in the diagnosis of dementia: Accuracy of diagnosis and consequences of misdiagnosis of disorders causing dementia. In R. D. Terry (Ed.), *Aging and the brain* (pp. 17–62). New York: Raven Press.

Lipowski, Z. J. (1983). Transient cognitive disorders (delirium, acute confusional states) in the elderly. *American Journal of Psychiatry, 140,* 1426–1436.

Mace, N., & Rabins, P. (1981). *The 36-hour day.* Baltimore, MD: John Hopkins University Press.

Mahendra, B. (1984). *Dementia: A survey of the syndrome of dementia.* Lancaster, UK: MTP Press.

McKeith, I. G., Galasko, D., Kosaka, K., Perry, E. K., Dickson, D. W., Hansen, L. A., Salmon, D. P., Lowe, J., Mira, S. S., Byrne, E. J., Lennox, G., Quinn, N. P., Edwardson, J. A., Ince, P. G., Beregron, C., Burns, A., Miller, B. L., Lovestone, S., Collerton, D., Jansen, E. N., Ballard, C., de Vos, R. A., Wilcock, G. K., Jellinger, K. A., & Perry, R. H. (1996). Consensus guidelines for the clinical and pathologic diagnosis of dementia with Lewy bodies (DLB): report of the consortium on DLS international workshop. *Neurology, 47,* 1113–1124.

Miller, B. L., Darby, A. L., Swartz, J. R., Yener, G. G., & Mena, I. (1995). Dietary changes, compulsions, and sexual behavior in frontotemporal degeneration. *Dementia, 6,* 195–199.

Progress Report on Alzheimer's Disease. (1998). Silver Spring, MD: ADEAR, National Institute on Aging.

Talbot, P. R. (1996). Frontal lobe dementia and motor neuron disease. *Journal of Neural Transmission* (Suppl.), 47, 125–132.

Taylor, A. E., Saint-Cyr, J. A., & Lang, A. E. (1986). Frontal lobe dysfunction in Parkinson's disease. *Brain, 109,* 845–883.

Thomas, C. L. (1981). *Taber's cyclopedic medical dictionary.* Philadelphia: F. A. Davis.

Torack, R. M. (1983). The early history of senile dementia. In B. Reisberg (Ed.), *Alzheimer's disease: The standard reference* (pp. 23–28). New York: Free Press.

U.S. Congress, Office of Technology Assessment. (1987). *Losing a million minds: Confronting the tragedy of Alzheimer's disease and other dementias.* Washington, DC: U.S. Government Printing Office.

Wells, C. E. (1979). Pseudodementia. *American Journal of Psychiatry, 136,* 898–900.

Wurtman, R. J. (1985). Alzheimer's disease. *Scientific American, 252,* 62–75.

P A R T I

COMMUNICATION ISSUES

Sensory and Communication Changes in Normal and Demented Elders

LEARNING OBJECTIVES

- To identify sensory changes accompanying aging
- To suggest how these sensory changes interfere with communication
- To list age-related changes in speech and language
- To outline the effects of brain damage on the ability to use language
- To empathize with the frustration of trying to communicate following the loss of language abilities

PRETEST

Place a "T" before true statements, an "F" before false statements, and a question mark before those you don't know.

___ 1. Older people can see just as well in the dark as younger people.

___ 2. Older people who are hard of hearing can hear higher pitched sounds best.

___ 3. A stroke can affect a person's ability to speak as well as understand language.

____ 4. Persons with Alzheimer's disease (AD) often have trouble thinking of the names of things when they are talking.

____ 5. Aphasia means a loss of the ability to use or understand spoken language.

____ 6. The sense of touch declines rapidly as we age.

____ 7. Persons with dementia may take a longer time than others to respond to a question.

____ 8. Sometimes persons who have had a stroke can hear your voice but can no longer make sense out of your words.

____ 9. A person with AD usually looks animated and expressive.

____ 10. The loss of the sense of smell can mean safety concerns for nursing home residents.

SENSORY CHANGES AND THEIR IMPACT

There are sensory changes that accompany aging in general and senile dementia in particular that interfere with interpersonal communication. These sensory changes may cause a person to show symptoms of dementia. They may also cause a person who is cognitively impaired to appear even more disabled. Awareness and understanding of these changes will help those who care for elderly people.

Changes in Vision

Vision is a very important sense. However, with aging there are common changes in vision. One of the changes in the eye that comes with age is the loss of elasticity of the lens of the eye. It is no longer able to focus or accommodate sufficiently for a person to clearly see material that is close to the eye. People usually begin to notice this in their 40s and will require corrective lenses in order to be able to read fine print (Goldman, 1979). Other changes in the eye include decreased pupil size, loss of lens transparency, and increased thickening of the capsule, all acting to reduce the amount of light that reaches the retina. Thus, more light must be available for the elderly person to be able to see (Storandt, 1986). Older people require lighting three or four

Answers: 1-F, 2-F, 3-T, 4-T, 5-T, 6-F, 7-T, 8-T, 9-F, 10-T.

times brighter than younger people in order to be able to see clearly (Brawley, 1997; Kenney, 1988). However, older people's eyes are also more susceptible to glare, so they often avoid bright light that would help their visual acuity (Storandt, 1986). Also, tiny bits of debris accumulate in the lens that reflect light and produce a glare that is very bothersome and distracting.

Because the pupil of the eye (which regulates the amount of light that gets into the eye) becomes rigid and fixed with age, older people have more difficulty adjusting to sudden changes in the level of lighting. Their eyes do not adjust as rapidly as those of younger people when they move from a light to a dark area or vice versa (Kenney, 1988). Some residents are even afraid to venture from their rooms, as the hallway looks dark and perhaps scary to them.

Mr. Evans always dreaded leaving his well-lit room for the dim hallway and would bump into carts and other residents as he walked down the corridor.

Residents may have difficulty finding seats in the dark recreation room during movies, so they show up very early and find seats well in advance of a movie showing.

With age, the fluid in the front part of the eye begins to turn yellow. This affects a person's ability to discriminate colors, especially to tell the difference between blues and greens. That is why a sign with green print on a blue background might not be understood by residents. Older adults may wear clothing with clashing colors or food spots. This may be interpreted as a sign of inattention to self-care or even dementia. However, it may be instead a result of their inability to discriminate colors correctly (Saxon & Etten, 1994). Reds and yellows are usually perceived best (Phillips, 1981).

Diseases of the eye, such as cataracts, glaucoma, macular degeneration, and visual problems secondary to stroke or diabetes, become more common as one grows older. Cataracts occur when the lens of the eye becomes cloudy, making vision difficult. It has been said that if people lived to be 120 or 130 years old, everybody would have cataracts (Kenney, 1988). Cataracts can be removed surgically, and the person's vision will usually be significantly improved.

Glaucoma is a disease causing increased pressure within the eye that can damage the structure of the eye and impair vision. It can be treated with medication. Macular degeneration accounts for most of the new cases in acquired adult legal blindness in the United States

(Anderson, 1987). The condition results when the focus point of the retina, the fovea, degenerates so that it can no longer function. Peripheral vision is maintained, but the individual can not see well enough to read or drive a car. A stroke may cause damage to the centers in the brain that control vision—although the eye can see, the brain cannot interpret images. Diabetes can lead to disruptions in blood flow to the retina, and is another leading cause of blindness in the later years (Anderson, 1987). By controlling diabetes, eye changes as a result of diabetes may be prevented. Also, laser photocoagulation may be useful in preventing or slowing visual loss if signs of diabetic changes to the retina are discovered early enough (Saxon & Etten, 1994).

These diseases provide a serious threat to the vision of the elderly. Having one of these diseases can lead an older person to become more dependent on those around them. Disease affecting vision, along with the normal changes in the aging eye, can interfere with a person's ability to read or watch television. This cuts down on the amount of information an older person can take in from the outside world. These changes also affect a person's ability to move around freely. Aside from no longer being able to drive a car, visual problems make a person reluctant to leave a familiar house or room to venture into the unknown. People with visual problems can feel very disoriented, uncertain, and isolated. Communication can also be affected by poor vision, as the elder can't see your lips or facial expressions.

If the person also has dementia, both the visual and the cognitive problems will be worsened. As a result of the dementia, the person will be less able to learn new habits to compensate for these visual changes. The disorientation and uncertainty resulting from vision loss will exacerbate those same feelings resulting from dementia, leading to an excess disability.

Changes in Hearing

Changes in hearing that accompany aging are even more important for interpersonal communication than changes in vision. The change in hearing that most typically occurs with increasing age is called presbycusis. It is a progressive hearing loss in both ears that is the result of sensorineural changes (Phillips, 1981). Men are more likely to suffer this loss than women, possibly because they have been more exposed to higher levels of noise over long periods of time in their work environment (Saxon & Etten, 1994). Hearing of higher frequencies, or higher pitched sounds, is particularly affected. For example, women's higher voices are more difficult to hear than men's lower voices. Sound discrimination is also affected. Consonants such as s, z, t, f, and g may be very hard for the older person to discriminate. These particular consonants are spoken at a higher pitch and with very little power behind them (Storandt, 1986). After age 60, there is some decline in the understanding of speech, and by age 80 there is a 25% loss in the discrimination of speech sounds (Benjamin, 1988; Corso, 1987). Older people also have a particularly difficult time understanding speech if there is a lot of background noise.

It is obvious that these changes in hearing ability might make it very difficult for older persons to understand what is being said to them. Not hearing the higher pitched sounds and not hearing important consonants could make some conversations almost impossible to understand, especially in a noisy background.

Mrs. Ables baffled the staff at the nursing home. When they would talk to her, she would repeat back some very strange and unusual words and sounds as if trying to make sense out of what she heard them saying. They thought she might have dementia, but after an audiology consult, it was discovered that she had severe hearing loss.

Many caregivers are women who naturally have higher pitched voices than men. Also, when we are talking with someone who is hard of hearing, we automatically raise our voices in pitch as well as volume. Our natural reaction to help someone hear actually makes it harder for them to hear. The solution is to consciously lower the pitch of your voice and to speak clearly at a normal speed while facing the person to whom you are talking. Many elderly people naturally pick up some lip-reading abilities to enhance their ability to understand what is being said to them. They also show an increased sensitivity to loud noises, so speaking too loudly to them may be counterproductive. The loudness makes them want to withdraw rather than listen. It is common to hear an older person say, "You don't have to yell!" when you have simply raised your voice slightly in order to be understood. As mentioned earlier, older people have greater difficulty hearing what is said to them when there is a high level of background noise. When the television is blaring, a vacuum cleaner is running in the hall, and there are announcements coming over the public address system, it might be better to wait for a quieter time to get an important message across.

There are several typical reactions to having a hearing loss. One reaction is to withdraw and give up trying to interact with others because it is so frustrating and unsatisfying. Another reaction is to become irritable and annoyed with everyone because they are "mumbling" or "not speaking clearly." The television is too soft, while everyone else complains that it is too loud. This kind of denial can lead to constant friction and bickering with others and makes life generally unpleasant. A third reaction to hearing impairment is to become suspicious of what others are saying and doing. Hearing impaired people see other people talking in what is thought to be a whisper and assume they are talking about them. In fact, families and other caregivers of hearing impaired persons often do get in the habit of talking in their presence as if they weren't there. Hard of hearing persons who are paranoid about what is being said about them can become very bitter and angry about the situation and feel helpless to control their own fate.

Mr. Barry had profound hearing loss to which he would never admit. He began to think his neighbor across the hall was out to get him. He would drag heavy furniture in front of his door at night so that no one could open it. After receiving a hearing aid, Mr. Barry's hearing improved somewhat, and he became much less paranoid. He even began to talk with his neighbor.

People who have difficulty hearing also often get in the habit of agreeing with others even when they have not heard what has been said. This can be a problem for caregivers who think the person knows what was said when actually the person does not. One way to ensure that important information has been communicated to the hard of hearing person is to ask the person to repeat back what was just said.

When a person has dementia and is also hard of hearing, communication is doubly difficult. The difficulty in comprehending language that often accompanies dementia is compounded by hearing difficulties. These problems can be truly isolating and lead the person to withdraw and want to avoid social contact. Attempts to improve hearing with hearing aids are worthwhile but usually require some persistence on the part of the caregiver. Hearing aids require considerable motivation to learn to use and to overcome initially unpleasant sensations of wearing them along with the distortions of sound they introduce (Phillips, 1986). Demented persons often lack the motivation to tolerate and overcome these unpleasant sensations. Also, they will not remember they have a hearing aid or that they need to change the batteries. The caregiver often must take the daily responsibility of reminding the patient to wear the hearing aid, turn it on, clean it of ear wax, change the batteries as needed, and keep it in a safe place when not being worn. The reward is that when demented persons can hear what is going on around them, they will be less confused, feel less isolated, take a greater part in social events, and have a more fulfilled life.

Changes in Taste and Smell

Aging also results in changes in the sharpness of the senses of taste and smell. While these senses are less directly involved with interpersonal communication, the loss of these senses can lead to a decreased quality of life for the resident, which could contribute to depression and apathy.

Taste

Studies show that there is some decline in taste sensitivity with age, although it is a relatively small change (Storandt, 1986). However, such habits as smoking, chewing tobacco, heavy alcohol use, or poor oral care can greatly increase this loss of sensitivity. This is unfortunate, as eating and mealtimes are opportunities for socialization and pleasure. When taste is decreased, people complain about their food or stop eating, which interferes with positive experiences during mealtimes.

Smell

In general, studies have found there is a decline in the functioning of the sense of smell with age (Schiffman, 1987). Older people have been found to perceive smells as less intense than do younger people. Older people also show a decreased ability to identify odors. They have also been found to be more tolerant of unpleasant odors. Again, smoking, the use of certain medications, and some illnesses can accelerate the losses in olfactory sensitivity in older adults.

Several studies have noted that persons with Alzheimer's disease are more likely than other older adults to suffer a loss of the sense of smell. The deficits occur in the recognition of smells as well as in the threshold at which a smell is perceived (Coffey & Cummings, 1994; Katzman et al., 1988). In persons with AD, senile plaques, neurofibrillary tangles, and cell loss have been found in the brain's olfactory areas (Schiffman, 1987) which probably account for the impairment in the sense of smell.

The loss of this sense, perhaps more than deficits in the sense of taste, can affect the eating habits of older adults. Most of what we commonly refer to as "taste" in food depends on our sense of smell to discriminate the flavors. Impairment in the ability to distinguish the flavors in foods can lead to several problems. One problem is that the pleasure received from eating and food-related activities such as cooking is diminished. If eating is less pleasurable, loss of appetite and lack of interest in eating often follow. This can be a particular problem for a person with dementia who may not have the judgment to be aware of the importance of eating and may even forget whether or not a meal has been eaten. Such a lack of interest in food can lead to malnutrition and dehydration. These are significant health risks in the elderly and can lead to increased dementia, if not death.

Another safety issue involved with the decreased sensitivity of the sense of smell is that such an impairment affects the ability to sense danger. The greater tolerance older people show of unpleasant odors suggests that they may not perceive the danger of gas leaks, smoke, or other odors that serve as a warning. Thus, they might be less likely to quickly seek safety when in a dangerous situation. Also, with an inability to distinguish the flavors of foods, the individual might overlook the bad taste of a spoiled or contaminated food item, increasing the risk for food poisoning (Kenney, 1988). The caregiver needs to be aware of these deficits older people experience in taste and smell. Smoke detectors should be in place in all living situations, and the refrigerator should be cleaned out frequently. Demented individuals also have a tendency to hoard food in their clothes and drawers. These must be routinely checked as well.

Tolerating unpleasant odors can also affect older persons' hygiene. If they cannot smell their own body odor, they may not realize that they need to bathe. This can make interactions very unpleasant and can cause a battle at bath time.

Sense of Touch

The sense of touch is a complicated sense. It includes the perception of pressure, vibration, temperature, pain, the position of the body in space, and the localization of a touch (Phillips, 1981). What you feel is usually in interaction of these touch processes. Studies suggest that there is a general decrease in touch sensitivity in older people, but less than 50% of the older people tested showed this decrease (Phillips, 1981). The decrease in touch sensitivity is most pronounced in the feet and becomes less apparent as you move up the body toward the head. This greater impairment in the feet and lower extremities mainly applies to perception of vibration and position of the feet. This may lead to increased danger of falling or tripping over things. Hands may also be affected, causing an increase in the dropping of objects.

Older people appear to be able to detect changes in temperature about as well as younger people. However, older people seem to have more difficulty adjusting to extremes of temperature. This suggests impairment of their internal regulating system but not their temperature sense.

Older people are more likely to have medical problems that lead to impairments in the sense of touch. Persons with dementia are known to have an impaired vibratory sense. Also, strokes, diabetic and peripheral neuropathies, and other conditions prevalent in old age affect the sense of touch.

Despite the evidence of impairment in this sense, however, touch is the sense that basically remains functioning when other senses have become blunted by age or disease. As such, touch becomes an extremely important way to communicate with otherwise impaired residents. Touch can be used to gain a person's attention, to reassure, to let the person know you are there to help, or to guide the person in some activity.

Touch is a very powerful therapeutic tool. Older people are very touch deprived—they are less touched than other age groups in medical settings, and have less opportunities for touch from family members and friends after relocation to nursing homes. The touch of the caregiver is therefore that much more important. Realize, however, that some individuals do not enjoy the touch of others and may react negatively to an unwelcome approach (Saxon & Etten, 1994). One must gauge the reactions of the particular resident. Perhaps over time the resident will come to trust the caregiver and enjoy a gentle massage or handclasp.

Sensory Deprivation

With the impairment of sight and hearing, along with restriction of movement and strength that illness imposes, many older people are at risk for sensory deprivation. The brain appears to require a certain minimal amount of sensory input to remain alert and functioning. Severe sensory impairments can lead to sensory deprivation, which sometimes results in behavior similar to dementia or psychosis. A person who cannot see or hear well and is also suffering from dementia may become even more disoriented and confused. When this person's world is further restricted by being confined to bed or gerichair for long periods, with little to indicate the passage of time or circumstances of their environment, the deprivation of sensory stimulation is even more complete. Many repetitive problem behaviors, such as chanting, pounding rhythmically on the chair or bed, picking at or scratching the skin may be responses to the lack of sensory stimulation. Hallucinations are another possible response. People engaging in such behaviors are trying to create their own stimulation, since there is no stimulation that they can perceive around them.

Touch can be used to provide sensory stimulation for people with severe sensory impairments of vision and hearing. You can use touch—different textures, massage, a guiding hand—to improve orientation or to provide an "anchor in reality" and the stimulation necessary to keep the person alert and functioning (Phillips, 1981). Participation in cognitive stimulation groups, often run by occupational therapists, can also be helpful. One enjoyable exercise is to use "scratch and sniff" cards with different smells such as flowers, popcorn, baked goods, etc. The planned use of music, including having the resident play drums or bells, can provide important sensory experiences even for hearing impaired individuals. Also, varying the visual landscape with different objects, posters, and fabrics of contrasting colors can provide visual stimulation for all but the totally blind. A trip outdoors can offer stimulation to all the senses. Other sensory stimulation best practices are described by Hoffman (1998).

Changes in Facial Expression

An impairment that often accompanies Alzheimer's disease, Parkinson's disease, and vascular dementia and that interferes with interpersonal communication is a decrease in facial expressiveness (Heilman, Schwartz, & Watson, 1978). Persons with these disorders often have a "flat affect"—that is, their facial expression does not change much during emotional situations. It often seems that people with a flat affect have to use an excessive amount of effort to smile or otherwise change their expression. This interferes with interpersonal communication because we all depend on changes in the facial expressions of another to know if what we are saying is being heard and understood. We are rewarded for our efforts in talking to someone by having that person smile at appropriate places and otherwise react facially to what is being said. When persons do not respond to what we say with changes in their facial expression, it becomes frustrating and less rewarding to talk to them. We may have a tendency to avoid them or not bother trying to talk to them any longer. This avoidance can lead to further apathy and withdrawal in dementia residents.

Although facial expression may be limited, the authors in a key study have found that sensitivity to the nonverbal cues of others is preserved (Hoffman, Platt, Barry, & Hamill, 1985). Though less expressive themselves, residents are still responding to nonverbal expressiveness in others. For example, when caregivers frown, residents know the caregivers are upset, which can in turn upset the residents.

Speech and Language Changes and Their Impact

The use of language is extremely important in our day-to-day functioning. There are speech and language changes that accompany normal aging. Also, with impairment of brain functioning either through head injury, a stroke, or AD, there is often a decrease in the ability to use language.

When you hear the voice of a stranger over the telephone, you usually have some mental image of the age of the individual. We all can identify voices as young or old and will usually be correct. There are systematic changes in the structure and tissues involved in voice production as we age. These changes include muscle atrophy, reduction in muscle strength and tissue elasticity, and reduction in breathing efficiency, which are all sufficient to alter the speaking voice (Benjamin, 1988). Older voices are also lower in pitch than younger voices and have a slight hoarseness (Cavannaugh, 1996). Older speakers also apparently lose some ability to vary the pitch of their voices and show an increase in voice tension when they speak. Many of these changes are influenced by the physical condition of the speaker, including the presence or absence of teeth. Very limited changes are noted in the voices of healthy older adults. One effect of the changes in voice of older adults is that others respond to these changes in stereotypical ways. For example, one might find oneself speaking louder to all older people, even if they don't have a hearing problem. We also tend to use simpler language with older people, and then think to ourselves that they, therefore, must be simple people. It is important to guard against these stereotypes and relate to each older adult as an individual.

Perhaps more significant than changes in the voice of older persons are changes in the older person's ability to articulate sounds clearly and a slowing in the rate of speech (Benjamin, 1988). In addition to the changes in speech production, there are changes in the way people use language as they age. Many of these changes are related to age-associated sensory changes, memory, and thinking abilities (Ryan, 1991). Older adults are more likely to have word-finding difficulties, and their speech may be less smooth with more hesitations. They may be less able to effectively get across information or ask appropriate questions than younger adults. However, it has been found that older adults excel in such conversational skills as taking conversational turns, finding common areas of interest with their partners, changing topics smoothly, and adapting their communication style to the needs of their partners (Benjamin, 1988). It seems that years of experience and practice in conversing with others pays off in better conversational skills in later years.

Communication Disorders

Older people are at increased risk for several types of communication disorders primarily because of their higher risk of having strokes, dementia, and other disorders of the central nervous system that affect speech and language. These communication disorders include aphasia, dysarthrias, and other communication deficits associated with impaired brain functioning.

Aphasia

Aphasia is a general term meaning a reduction in the ability to use or understand language as a result of brain damage (Obler & Albert, 1980; Tonkonvich, 1988). Depending on the area of the brain damaged, there can be different problems in the use of language. The temporal and parietal lobes of the brain are mainly affected when language is impaired (see Figure 1.1). A person who has a stroke and is paralyzed on the right side of the body often also has speech problems as a result of the stroke. This is because right-sided paralysis indicates that the

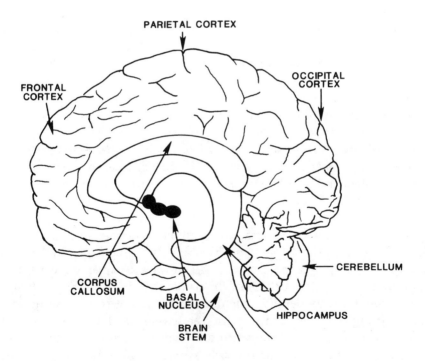

FIGURE 1.1   Identification of brain areas.

stroke occurred on the left side of the brain, and for most people, language centers are located in the left brain hemisphere. (The "l" in both "left" and "language" will help recall on which side of the brain the language centers are usually located.)

A person who suffers damage toward the front of the brain's left hemisphere may have damage in a speech center called "Broca's area." People with damage in this area understand what you say to them fairly well and know what they want to say, but they can't make the words come out right. This is referred to as Broca's or expressive aphasia and can be very frustrating to the person experiencing it. Interestingly enough, the individual may be able to speak a few words clearly, such as curse words, and may be able to sing. The use of a personalized communication book is usually very helpful to a person with this problem—the book contains words and sentences that this particular person often uses. The resident can point to certain phrases in the book in order to communicate something.

Persons who suffer damage farther toward the back of the brain in the region called "Wernicke's area" may be fairly fluent in their speech, but they don't understand what you say to them, and what they say doesn't make much sense. This is called Wernicke's or receptive aphasia. Stroke victims may have predominantly expressive aphasia or predominantly receptive aphasia, or even both kinds of aphasia together, depending on the site and extent of the brain lesion.

Two other types of aphasia often seen in older adults are global aphasia and anomic aphasia. These aphasias are caused by more widespread damage to the brain (Tonkovich, 1988). Global aphasia involves severe impairments in all areas of language. Speech is sparse and meaningless and people understand little that is said to them.

Persons with anomic aphasia or anomia show an inability to produce the names of objects when asked what they are and have word-finding problems in general conversation. "Anomia" is derived from the Greek words "a" meaning without and "onomos" meaning name. Individuals with anomic aphasia may use roundabout ways of explaining what they mean when they can't think of the name of something. For instance, a person asked to identify a picture of a bat might reply "a thing that flies at night." They also may use the wrong word, or they may just give up trying to find the word and continue with what they were saying. Anomia is a common early symptom of Alzheimer's disease. Caregivers can help supply the correct word. However, some individuals with dementia prefer to try to find the word themselves, while others appreciate this help. Asking questions that can be answered by "yes" or "no" may also be helpful to improve communication.

Right Brain Hemisphere Damage

Persons who have strokes in the right hemisphere of the brain (left-sided paralysis) have more subtle problems with their speech. They usually are able to talk fairly well. However, the deficits tend to show up in conversational speech. Problems appear in organizing conversation, distinguishing between important and unimportant details, staying on the topic, and being sensitive to the situation and the other participants in the conversation (Tonkovich, 1988). Thus, persons with right hemisphere damage are apt to show deficits in the very conversational skills in which, as mentioned previously, older people generally do very well.

Dysarthria

Dysarthria is a motor speech disorder in which brain damage has led to muscle weakness and/or involuntary movements that impair speech production and result in slurred speech (Tonkovich, 1988). The person has difficulty physically forming words or making words flow smoothly because of difficulty controlling muscles of the jaw, tongue, throat, etc. This is not the same as aphasia. Persons with dysarthria can easily understand verbal communication. Many disorders affecting the brain can cause dysarthria. These include stroke or multi-infarcts, tumors, toxic or metabolic disorders, Parkinson's disease, amyotrophic lateral sclerosis, multiple sclerosis, and Wilson's disease (Tonkovich, 1988). Dysarthrias result from damage in the subcortical areas of the brain. They are not an early sign of progressive cortical dementing illness such as AD, but may occur late in the course of a cortical dementia when subcortical areas also become affected (Campbell-Taylor, 1991).

Other Dementia-Related Communication Problems and Solutions

There are other problems with verbal communication seen in persons with dementia. One problem is they become very "concrete" in their thinking—no longer able to understand abstractions. Thus, if you are speaking to them in an indirect, abstract way, they may misinterpret what you say or just not understand. *For instance, Mrs. Cook did not understand when her nurse said her room was "just down the hall."* "Down" taken literally refers to a vertical direction, rather than a horizontal direction. Our language is full of abstractions and metaphors that can be very disconcerting to a person with dementia. The busy caregiver might be tempted to remark, "Can't you see I'm all tied up?" Of course, this would not be understood.

Another problem in verbal communication with dementia patients is the delayed reaction time they typically show in conversation with someone. We have learned to expect a response to a question or comment within a very short period of time, usually a few seconds or less. If a person does not respond within that timeframe, you can usually tell by the facial expression that the person is thinking of an answer. When interacting with persons with dementia who may have a nonexpressive face and a delayed response time, we often think they haven't heard us or are not going to answer, and so we go on to the next question. Sometimes their response to your next question is actually their answer to your first question. This can lead to very confusing communications.

The memory problems of dementia residents also interfere with communication in that they often forget what was just said to them or what they were in the middle of saying. They might lose their train of thought in the middle of a sentence or even forget the end of the word they were trying to say. "Pancake" might come out "pan. . . . " Recognition problems also cause conversational confusion. If the dementia resident thinks you are a daughter rather than the nurse, questions may be answered very differently.

Mr. Adams thought the psychologist interviewing him was an insurance salesman, and he answered her questions as if she were a persistent salesperson.

Another conversational problem is the perseveration of persons with dementia—they get stuck on a subject, or just keep repeating themselves over and over. Persons with AD may also demonstrate echolalia—repeating what was just said to them, but not responding to the statement or question.

As the dementia progresses, language difficulties become progressively more severe. However, the person with dementia may have some good days, where recognition, memory, and language are somewhat improved.

Communication techniques that can enhance the interaction between resident and caregiver include using very simple and repetitive language and reliance on more nonverbal means of communicating. When speaking with a resident, short sentences and yes/no questions are helpful. If the person doesn't initially understand, repeat yourself exactly. If the person still can't understand, say the message another way. Nonverbal communication can be effective. This means having a calm and soothing approach, using gestures, and having a friendly facial expression. A communication book prepared by a speech pathologist may be useful. An understanding and a positive attitude is also helpful—allowing time for responding, and expecting perseveration. A good sense of humor is always important—without, of course, making fun of residents. Dementia residents also find movement and music to be very enjoyable. Singing songs with residents, dancing to an old tune, and encouraging their participation in group exercise programs is helpful. And of course, just holding a hand or giving a warm hug shows concern.

Communicating with persons with impaired language abilities can be very frustrating and discouraging for both parties involved (Wilder & Weinstein, 1984). It is also difficult to talk with someone who is very hard of hearing. You may have had experiences in trying to understand what is wrong with someone who isn't able to use language effectively but is obviously in distress (e.g., your young baby, an individual with a stroke). Think about the feelings such encounters can arouse—frustration, pity, sadness, a sense of loneliness. In this way, you can get a better appreciation of the problems of impaired communication. The speech pathologist or occupational therapist can be consulted for alternative strategies for communication.

SUMMARY

There are changes in vision, hearing, taste, smell, and touch that naturally accompany aging. In addition, there are changes in communication abilities that accompany age, dementia, and other diseases. All these changes lead to difficulties in maintaining independence, emotional well-being, and quality of life. The caregiver must be aware of these changes and alert to the difficulties and dangers these changes can present to an elderly person. Strategies can be developed so that communication can be maintained and the older person can continue to have a rewarding life (see Table 1.1).

LEARNING EXERCISES

1. Sensory loss simulation exercise
    a. Supplies needed: plastic sandwich bags, cotton balls, tongue depressors, tape
    b. Preparation: Tape plastic sandwich bags over eyeglasses or to forehead to simulate vision loss. Place moistened cotton balls (excess water squeezed out) in ears to simulate hearing loss. Tape tongue depressors to fingers or across knee joints to simulate stiffness of arthritis.
    c. Activities to try while disabled:
       • Read notices posted on bulletin board or signs.
       • Get a drink of water.
       • Identify or open a medicine bottle.
       • Select and eat a snack.
       • Look up a phone number in a book and make the call.
       • Take a walk outside of the room, and bring back several objects (e.g., pencil stone, leaf, etc.
       • Have a five-minute conversation with another person.
    d. Reactions
       • What losses did you simulate?
       • What activities did you try to do?
       • What were your thoughts and feelings during the experience?
       • What did you learn about yourself and others?
       • Do you have a better appreciation for the changes and coping strategies of older adults?
2. Think of experiences you have had where you needed to communicate with someone but were unable to because of barriers in the communication.
    a. Examples
       • Someone who only speaks and understands a foreign language that you don't know.
       • Someone who is very hard of hearing.

TABLE 1.1   Sensory Changes and How to Help

Sense system	Change	How to help
Vision	1) Lens becomes rigid, can't adjust for near/far vision	1) Bifocals
	2) Color discrimination decreases	2) Vivid colors
	3) Sensitivity to glare increases	3) Low glare lights
	4) Pupil reaction time slowed	4) Night lights
	5) Eye requires more light	5) Higher intensity lighting/ low glare bulbs; increased use of natural light
	6) Decreased range of vision	6) Approach from front
Hearing	1) Loss of ability to hear high frequency sounds	1) Lower pitch of voice
	2) Increased sensitivity to loud noises	2) Do not raise voice
	3) Decreased ability to hear above background noise	3) Reduce background noise, e.g., turn off television
	4) Decreased hearing due to an increase in ear wax	4) Check ears frequently for hardened ear wax, and clean it out properly
Taste/Smell	1) Decreased sensitivity of taste leading to poor food intake and enjoyment	1) Increase intensity of food flavors
	2) Decreased sensitivity of smell leading to inability to perceive dangerous stimuli	2a) Stimulate sense of smell with "scratch and sniff" cards
		2b) Use smoke detectors and increased caregiver vigilance
Touch	1) Decreased sensitivity in feet and hands can lead to accidents	1) Provide environment safe for walking
	2) With loss of other senses, touch sensations may be important to keep patient involved	2) Encourage caregivers to use more touch with their residents; offer back rubs and hand massage

- Someone who has had a stroke and has expressive aphasia.
- Someone with AD who cannot think of the names of things and is vague in what is said to you and doesn't seem to understand what you are saying.
- Someone who doesn't talk at all except for "yes" or "no."
  b. What were your feelings in these kinds of encounters?
  c. What was most frustrating about such interactions?
  d. What do you typically do to improve communication?
  e. What have you tried that seemed to work best?
3. Think of five common examples of phrases and metaphors in the English language that would be difficult for a demented resident to understand, e.g., "Your explanation is as clear as mud!"
4. Assess the room you are in, and discuss its good and bad features for an older resident with vision problems.

POSTTEST

Place a "T" before true statements, an "F" before false statements, and a question mark before those you don't know.

_____ 1. Residents with visual problems can feel disoriented and isolated.

_____ 2. An older person who is hard of hearing often can hear lower pitched sounds better.

_____ 3. Dementia due to sensory deprivation may occur when someone is blind, deaf, and has little touch stimulation.

_____ 4. Older people with hearing loss are unable to learn to lipread.

_____ 5. A person with AD may show little change in facial expression.

_____ 6. Dysathria is the same as aphasia.

_____ 7. Presbycusis means loss of vision.

_____ 8. One of the early symptoms of AD is word-finding problems known as anomia.

_____ 9. Sometimes if you wait long enough, a person with dementia will answer a question you thought the person was unable to answer.

_____ 10. We often tend to stereotype older people by speaking to all older persons in a loud voice.

REFERENCES

Anderson, B. (1995). Eye: Clinical issues. In G. L. Maddox (Ed.), *The encyclopedia of aging* (2nd ed., pp. 242–244). New York: Springer Publishing Co.

Benjamin, B. J. (1988). Changes in speech production and linguistic behaviors with aging. In B. B. Shadden (Ed.), *Communication, behavior, and aging: A sourcebook for clinicians* (pp. 162–181). Baltimore: Williams & Wilkins.

Brawley, E. C. (1997). *Designing for Alzheimer's disease: Strategies for better care environments.* New York: Wiley.

Campbell-Taylor, I. (1991). Motor speech changes. In R. Lubenski (Ed.), *Dementia and communication* (pp. 70–82). Philadelphia: D.C. Decker.

Cavannaugh, J. C. (1996). *Adult development and aging.* New York: Brooks/Cole.

Coffey, C. E., & Cummings, J. L. (1994). *The American Psychiatric Press textbook of geriatric neuropsychiatry.* Washington, DC: American Psychiatric Press.

Corso, J. F. (1987). Hearing. In G. L. Maddox (Ed.), *The encyclopedia of aging* (2nd ed., pp. 317–319). New York: Springer Publishing Co.

Goldman, R. (1979). Decline in organ function with age. In I. Rossman (Ed.), *Clinical geriatrics* (2nd ed., pp. 23–59). Philadelphia: J. B. Lippincott.

Heilman, K. M., Schwartz, H. D., & Watson, R. T. (1978). Hypoarousal in persons with the neglect syndrome and emotional indifference. *Neurology, 28,* 229–232.

Hoffman, S. B., et al. (1985). When language fails: Nonverbal communication abilities of the demented. In J. T. Hutton & A. D. Kenney (Eds.), *Senile dementia of the Alzheimer type* (pp. 49–64). New York: Alan R. Liss.

Hoffman, S. B. (1998). Innovations in behavior management (pp. 13–23). In M. Kaplan & and S. B. Hoffman (Eds.), *Behaviors in dementia: Best practices for successful management.* Baltimore, MD: Health Professions Press.

Katzman, R., Lasker, B., & Bernstein, N. (1988). Advances in the diagnosis of dementia: Accuracy of diagnosis and consequences of misdiagnosis of disorders causing dementia. In R. D. Terry (Ed.), *Aging and the brain* (pp. 17–62). New York: Raven Press.

Kenney, R. A. (1988). Physiology of aging. In B. B. Shadden (Ed.), *Communication, behavior, and aging: A sourcebook for clinicians* (pp. 58–78). Baltimore: Williams & Wilkins.

Answers: 1-T, 2-T, 3-T, 4-F, 5-T, 6-F, 7-F, 8-T, 9-T, 10-T.

Obler, L., & Albert, M. (1980). *Language and communication in the elderly.* Lexington: Lexington Books.

Phillips, L. R. F. (1981). Care of the client with sensori perceptual problems. In M. O. Wolanin & L. R. F. Phillips (Eds.), *Confusion: Prevention and care* (pp. 171–267). St. Louis: C. V. Mosby.

Ryan, H. B. (1991). Normal aging and language. In R. Lubenski (Ed.), *Dementia and communication* (pp. 84–97). Philadelphia: D.C. Decker.

Saxon, M. V., & Etten, J. J. (1994). The sensory systems. In *Physical change and aging* (pp. 72–104). New York: Tireseas Press.

Schiffman, S. S. (1987). Smell. In G. L. Maddox (Ed.), *The encyclopedia of aging* (2nd ed., pp. 618–619). New York: Springer Publishing Co.

Storandt, M. (1986). Psychological aspects of aging. In I. Rossman (Ed.), *Clinical geriatrics* (3rd ed., pp. 606–617). Philadelphia: J. B. Lippincott.

Tonkovich, J. D. (1988). Communication disorders in the elderly. In B. B. Shadden (Ed.), *Communication, behavior, and aging: A sourcebook for clinicians* (pp. 197–215). Baltimore, MD: Williams & Wilkins.

Wilder, C., & Weinstein, B. (1984). *Aging and communication: Problems in management.* New York: Haworth Press.

Chapter 2

Communication Strategies with Dementia Residents

LEARNING OBJECTIVES

- To understand that communication involves both what we say and how we say it
- To learn that nonverbal messages are conveyed by us without our awareness
- To identify the elements of nonverbal communication including touch, facial expression, eye contact, voice tone, posture, proxemics, and gesture
- To identify and use nonverbal elements of communication when interacting with residents
- To list the positive effects of nonverbal communication
- To identify resident needs more effectively by noticing their nonverbal messages
- To use good verbal and listening techniques for better resident care

---

PRETEST

Place a "T" before true statements, an "F" before false statements, and a question mark before those you don't know.

____ 1. People communicate best when they sit still, stare straight ahead, and speak slowly and carefully.

____ 2. People are not usually aware of the nonverbal messages they are sending.

____ 3. It is not good to touch residents except when performing personal care functions.

____ 4. If a staff member is upset with a resident, the staff member's face usually won't show it.

____ 5. Residents with severe senile dementia usually don't understand anything the staff say or do to them.

____ 6. A good way to find out if a dementia resident is done eating would be to say, "You don't want to eat any more; do you?"

____ 7. Once you learn how to look for nonverbal messages, you will understand exactly what residents are trying to express.

____ 8. An effective way to figure out what a resident is feeling is to use the technique of "feeling identification."

____ 9. We tend to screen out information in the environment that is not important to us.

____ 10. Knowing about a resident's personal history makes no difference in the ability to care for or understand the resident.

IMPORTANCE OF NONVERBAL COMMUNICATION

In communicating with others, the whole body is used to get a message across: words, facial expressions, voice tone, posture, eyes, gestures. Communication is both verbal—what we say, and nonverbal—how we say it. In fact, Argyle (1988) suggests that nonverbal signals are far more powerful than verbal ones for expressing how we feel about something. And Mehrabian (1971) proposes that almost 93% of communications occur through nonverbal messages.

However, we are usually so wrapped up in what we want to say verbally that we fail to realize that nonverbal communication is also a very powerful way to communicate with others (Northouse & Northouse, 1998). In fact, mimes can use nonverbal communication exclu-

---

Answers: 1-F, 2-T, 3-F, 4-F, 5-F, 6-F, 7-F, 8-T, 9-T, 10-F.

sively to convey a story. Examples of mimes include Marcel Marceau and the funny colorful circus clowns. Another good example of nonverbal communication is television—lots of action shows have very little dialogue, just dramatic music and plenty of activity. Something you can do to understand the power of nonverbal communication is to turn off the sound on your favorite soap opera. The story line can be followed fairly well. How? The actors' facial expressions, eye contact, posture, and gestures will convey a large amount of information. In fact, these are the elements of nonverbal communication: eye contact, posture, spatial position, gesture, and touch (Budd & Ruben, 1972). In addition, there is voice tone, the way in which you say something, loudly or softly, with a lilt or in a flat monotone, quickly or slowly.

When we communicate with others, how we speak is just as important as what we are saying verbally. So why don't we use nonverbal communication in a planned way? A speech is sometimes carefully planned and rehearsed, such as how to ask the boss for a raise, yet nonverbal actions are rarely as carefully planned. There are four major reasons why people don't effectively use nonverbal communication.

The first reason is that because we talk so much, we tend to believe that words are more important than actions. We think that it is quicker and easier to talk rather than touch, to explain rather than demonstrate. However, there is truth in the old saying, "A picture is worth a thousand words."

A second reason we don't pay more attention to nonverbal communication is that we don't even realize we are communicating nonverbally. We are often unaware of our posture, eyes, hand gestures, head movements, and facial expressions. Although actors receive much training in this aspect of communication and are very conscious of it, most of us are not trained to notice this component of our communication. How many times has a parent or family member said to you, "Stand up; you're slouching," when you didn't even realize it? How often has a good friend said, "You look tired," which made you notice that yes, in fact, you did feel very tired. A great deal of information about our moods and beliefs is conveyed through nonverbal communication when we don't even know it. This is not to say that we can't be trained to recognize this in ourselves—that is what this chapter covers.

The third reason that nonverbal communication is avoided is that it can involve touching. Some of us don't like to touch others. Why not? Some of our early experiences growing up have influenced us.

"Don't touch" is an expression drilled in by protective parents. Also, in our culture, touching is less common than in European countries such as Italy, for example (Howell & Vetter, 1985). Too, it isn't satisfying to touch people who are not pleasant to look at, smell bad, or have unclean clothes and skin. Although touching babies is something we might enjoy, touching diseased or elderly persons is something we might fear. Also, it is commonly thought that individuals with senile dementia can't respond to touch meaningfully. However, research by Hoffman et al. (1985) found that even extremely demented persons are still very responsive to touch, voice tone, and facial expression.

One additional reason that nonverbal communication is practiced so little is that we fear it is time-consuming. We are afraid that when we stop to talk with residents and really carefully listen to what they are saying, this could take time away from necessary tasks on the unit. The time it takes to listen to residents, focusing attention solely on them and their individual needs, is potentially stressful at the moment, but is necessary for building a trusting relationship (see Figure 2.1). In the long run, however, by developing that trusting and caring relationship, fewer time-consuming crises will arise with residents. One director of nursing at a nursing home always stops to talk with a resident, using the person's name, standing very close, making eye contact, and touching the person lightly on the hand or arm.

> I always stop when one of the patients wants me to. I know that now is important to them . . . I think we can't afford not to stop . . . What is a minute or two to me when it means so much to them? (Blondis & Jackson, 1982)

This particular administrator feels that by showing the resident that she cares, he or she will have fewer problems in the long run and demand less time from her nurses and aides. Of course, an administrator does not personally have the day-to-day responsibilities of an aide or nurse on a unit. However, a caregiver might find some time for warm, friendly interaction with residents while waiting for trays, taking them to physical therapy, or whenever there is a bit of free time.

Touch

One of the most effective ways to communicate nonverbally with others is through touch (Northouse & Northouse, 1998). Touch is

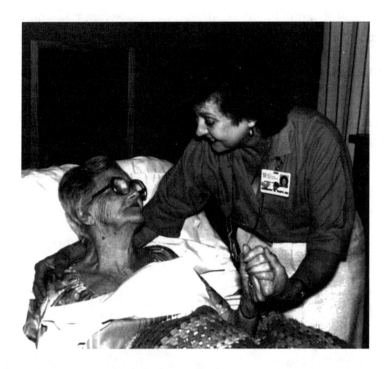

FIGURE 2.1   Focusing attention solely on resident, even for a short time, helps build a trusting relationship.

the earliest and most basic mode of communication (Montagu, 1971). Humans need touch for survival—early research from the 1950s determined that babies living in institutional settings who were not touched or held failed to thrive, and some even died. Touch is just as important to seriously ill and confused elderly individuals. It can calm and reassure the ill (McCorkle, 1974; Weiss, 1988) and can increase attention and nonverbal communication in the elderly confused (Langland & Panicucci, 1982). Bartol (1979) recommends touch to elicit listening on the part of residents and maintain his or her attention.

How the individual is touched is significant, as touch also can convey superior power and threat. DeWever (1977) found that nursing home residents prefer to be touched on the arm or face, rather than having nurses put an arm around their shoulders. Some female residents also felt discomfort when touched by male nurses.

Burnside (1973) advocates the "Indian handshake" in which you take the individual's hand and smother it between both of your hands (see Figure 2.2). If you try this, you will notice that you get a remarkably warm reception from the person. People seem to like having their hand held in this way. It is very reassuring to them, and it is a very caring gesture. Often, they will place another hand over yours.

What else can you do to increase touch? Another simple thing is to place your hand on the resident's arm or back while you are standing over the person, perhaps while waiting for meals to be served. Very often, caregivers touch the person's wheelchair handles, but they can't feel that. It would be much more comforting and really just as easy to touch their back or arm.

Some people, because of the way they were raised and their cultural values, feel uncomfortable when touched. Although gentle touch could probably benefit everyone, you might try to determine who doesn't want to be touched frequently. How can you tell? Simply through their nonverbal reactions to your touch. If people don't like being

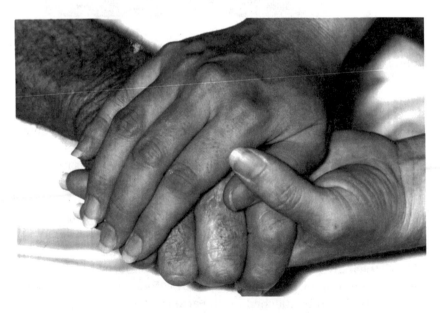

FIGURE 2.2   The Indian handshake: An example of nonverbal communication.

touched, they will probably withdraw. A resident may also say, "Don't touch me!"

Facial Expressions

There are six basic facial expressions: disgust, surprise, happiness, sadness, anger, and fear (Ekman, 1982). People often communicate one or a combination of these emotions without really knowing it, using forehead, eyebrows, nose, cheeks, skin color, and mouth to communicate facial emotions.

An important way to communicate better nonverbally is to understand what facial emotions are being conveyed to a person. This has been very simply stated: Know thyself. First, we must believe and understand that we really are communicating this information to others and that it is difficult if not impossible to hide our inner emotional reactions from those who know us. Residents will know when a caregiver is tired, irritable, didn't get enough sleep the last night, had a fight with a spouse or children, or feels impatient with them when they are slow.

Of course, we often try to hide our feelings from others. A caregiver may smile at a resident who is disliked. However, true feelings will sneak out—in very, very brief (less than two-fifths of a second) facial expressions called micromomentary expressions (Ekman, 1985). These brief facial expressions often "leak" or give away what a person is truly feeling. Also, if what you are saying disagrees with your facial expression, the listener will tend to believe your facial expression. Caregivers might say, "Now, this won't hurt a bit," while grimacing to themselves. Most people won't believe their words, because their face gives them away.

Because one can't really hide how one feels, it makes sense for caregivers to understand how they feel and to try to feel better about their residents. One may feel less impatient with demented residents knowing that because of brain damage, they really cannot stop themselves from behaving in annoying ways, such as moaning, scratching, or repeating phrases. Once a caregiver realizes that residents are picking up on impatient feelings and feeling bad themselves because of them, the caregiver can decide to try to feel better—by understanding the residents, getting more rest themselves, arguing less with family, getting more exercise, and feeling less stress.

Eye Contact

People tend to look at those they like and away from those they dislike (Ruffner & Burgoon, 1981). Eye contact is important during conversation, but it should be brief and often, rather than prolonged (like a stare). Looking at someone who is talking shows our interest in that person. Looking down or away conveys dislike, guilt, or boredom. Have you ever noticed a friend sneak a glance at a wristwatch while you were confiding in the person? Didn't you immediately feel rushed and upset?

Eyes can reveal our true feelings about someone. We can use them to help gain a person's trust and comfort. Early research (Hess & Holt, 1960) found that pupil size may indicate whether or not you like someone. When the pupil is enlarged, so that the eye looks darker, this can mean, among other things, that you like the person at whom you are gazing. If your pupil becomes smaller, this can mean you dislike that person.

The pupils in the eyes of the elderly are naturally smaller (Fozard et al., 1977). Older people often seem to have very light eyes with tiny pupils. We may unconsciously interpret this to mean that they don't like us. In defense, we may decide not to like them. We are not consciously aware of these very subtle dynamics. Often, we feel that we don't like or trust someone, yet can't figure out why. Knowledge such as this can make one aware of one's reaction to an older person's pupil size and prevent unconscious dislike.

Voice Tone

Voice tone, one aspect of paralanguage (Howell & Vetter, 1985), can be even more important than the words you are speaking. How you say something—your voice, pitch, rate, pauses, and silences—can reveal emotions behind your words.

One's voice tone, when providing care, is often very soothing and singsong—just the kind of voice tone parents use with very young infants. This is called baby talk or caretaker speech. Although a sooth-ing voice tone can be very effective with demented or aggressive residents, it may make someone who is only mildly demented feel "talked down to."

> *Mr. Robbins was eating lunch in the dining room, sitting apart from the rest of the residents. An aide walked in and cooed some nonsense syllables at him. He mumbled nonsense in return, appearing somewhat demented as he did this. Several minutes later, another aide came into the dining room and asked Mr. Robbins in a professional voice tone, "How did you enjoy your lunch?" He replied coherently, "It was quite good today."*

Caretakers need to monitor themselves and notice if they are using caretaker speech with all residents, or more appropriately, only with those who really respond best to it.

One excellent way to make use of voice tone is in calming an excited, anxious, or aggressive resident (Bartol, 1979). It is best for caregivers to approach this kind of person after taking a deep breath and calming themselves. Then in speaking to the individual, one should act nor-mally, lower the pitch of the voice, and speak slowly and soothingly. When someone is upset, it is very difficult for that person to take in new information. Therefore, the caregiver must speak slowly and perhaps repeat what he or she is saying several times. As he or she is talking slowly and soothingly, one can also take the resident away from the upsetting environment. A change of scene can help the residents forget what it was that caused them to get upset (because of their short-term memory loss).

Posture, Proxemics, and Gesture

Posture can also reveal how you are feeling about a person (Ekman & Friesen, 1969). Do your shoulders creep up high around your ears throughout the day? This occurs during stress. Remember to notice the tension in your shoulders, and relax them down. A closed posture (folding the arms in front of the body) can indicate dislike for a person and a need to protect oneself from them. An open posture, where the arms are relaxed down or are spread wide, can welcome the residents' approach (Fast, 1970). Of course, these postures can also be misinter-preted. Arms folded in front can mean simply that one is feeling cold.

Does the caregiver lean forward to listen to residents? This indicates interest in what they have to say. Do the caregivers nod their heads slightly every so often? This also shows that they are really listening (Danish & Hauer, 1977).

Where one stands is equally important. Caregivers often have to get very close to a person when providing personal care. This invades personal space, an imaginary bubble we all have around us (Hall, 1966). Penetrating this space, usually reserved for intimate acts with those we trust, can make residents feel very uncomfortable unless caregivers talk with them and explain what they are doing. When intimate space is violated, the individual tries to back up, turn away, or in some fashion withdraw from the encounter for protection. Residents may indeed have a severe reaction to sudden intrusions on their space, known as catastrophic reaction.

Residents with vision and hearing problems often can't see or hear the caregiver approach. Then suddenly a hand looms in on them and frightens them. It is best to approach slowly, at their eye level if possible, and announce oneself in advance. Nurses and aides often have to interact with residents in bed or wheelchairs. It is easy to approach from the back or side. However, this can startle a person. An approach from the front is best, bending or squatting down to be at eye level.

Gestures are another important aspect of body language. If someone can't understand a person's words because of a problem with aphasia, dementia, or hearing loss, they may understand a gesture. Gestures can help others understand the content and emotions of one's words. A hug means I like you. A smile means I feel friendly toward you. Most of us naturally gesture as we talk, some of us more than others. It is helpful to consciously use gesture to convey a message. If residents don't understand a caregiver's words, the meaning should be conveyed with gesture. For instance, if a resident won't respond when a caregiver says, "It's time for your pill," the caregiver should say the resident's name and then pretend to take a pill, and pretend to drink a glass of water.

UNDERSTANDING THE NONVERBAL MESSAGES OF RESIDENTS WITH DEMENTIA

Although demented individuals may have impaired verbal communication abilities, they still are able to communicate nonverbally (Bartol,

1979; Preston, 1973). Through careful observation, nonverbal behaviors can be used to understand residents better—how they are feeling and what they may need. Because dementia residents will have limitations in verbal communication, it is important to give them the opportunity to express themselves as freely as possible. By sitting or standing at the person's eye level with an open body posture, leaning forward to show interest, and by making eye contact to show liking for the person, caregivers will convey caring and the willingness to listen. Because of this trust building, residents will feel more secure and comfortable about openly expressing their feelings and needs. They will also be more willing to comply with requests and instructions.

Although we take in tremendous amounts of information all the time, most of this data is screened out by the reticular activating system of the brain. Usually, we screen out things that don't interest us. How often do you notice the make and model of all the cars on the road? But imagine you are planning to buy a new car and aren't sure of which type you want. Suddenly cars are interesting to you, and you begin to avidly watch cars on the road. In the same manner, if caregivers remind themselves to use the information they are taking in to evaluate the resident's physical and emotional well-being, they will become much better observers. One can use the many small cues that usually go unobserved in everyday resident care to notice when a resident is experiencing an infection, or even a heart attack, or maybe just feels lonely or depressed. Residents may become happier too as they receive more attention. As their emotional well-being improves, they may be easier to manage and care for. Thus, there are many benefits, both for the caregivers and residents, to becoming more careful observers. It is useful to observe residents' facial expressions, eyes, gesturing, and vocalizations.

Facial Expressions

As discussed previously, individuals with dementia may no longer be as animated in their facial expressiveness as they once were. The face may appear to be rigid, almost as if it were a mask. But if one looks closely and carefully, one may be able to see some small changes which can give an indication of the emotions the resident may be experiencing. Ekman (1982) suggests that eyebrows, eyes, nose, and mouth are used to convey the six basic emotions of happiness, sadness, surprise, fear, anger, and disgust. Blondis and Jackson (1982) describe these facial expressions as follows: with happiness, lower eyelids crinkle, cheeks are raised, the mouth smiles. With sadness, the face droops or appears slack, and the mouth may tremble. Surprise is a very fleeting facial expression—the eyebrows arch high, eyes open wide, and the jaw drops. With fear the eyebrows rise up and draw together, eyes are open and tensed, and lips are stretched back. Anger is expressed by lowered, drawn eyebrows, staring eyes, and a rigid mouth. And disgust is mainly expressed through a wrinkled nose and raised upper lip.

Eyes

Although the face may become more rigid and affect may appear flat, the eyes may show that the person is still aware, can understand things to some extent, and can give an indication of emotion with eyebrows, eyelids, and change in pupil size. Some things to look for include widening or narrowing of the eyes, eye movement, tension in the lids, and tearing of the eyes.

Tears can be an indication of extreme emotion in the elderly. They mean happiness, fear, or sadness; however, they can also be a signal of emotional lability that comes with certain dementing illnesses. We all need to cry in order to express our grief and ultimately recover from it. Certainly, dementia residents have much to mourn—not only the loss of their homes, their families, and their jobs, but also an essential part of themselves—their personality and reasoning. In addition, because of memory loss, dementia residents may also freshly mourn a long-dead relative.

It is difficult to be around someone who is crying. Caregivers might be tempted to try to cheer up the residents. However, it is far better to acknowledge their grief and let them cry themselves out. One should simply give the person a tissue, hold her hand, and say, "It's okay to cry."

Lack of eye contact from demented residents may mean they are not ready or willing to listen.

If you do not have the ADT patient's undivided listening attention, you cannot be assured that he has heard or understood what you have said, nor are you

assured of compliance. Nonlistening behavior is characterized by lack of direct
eye contact, the patient's body position faced away from the nurse. (Bartol, 1979)

The emotion and intelligence sometimes expressed in the eyes of
residents who can no longer talk or understand tells us that there is
still the soul of a human being residing within dementia residents,
human beings who deserve caring and respect. As one looks into a
resident's eyes, and he or she looks back, the eye contact may help
one feel that some awareness is truly there, even in the most advanced
stages of a dementing illness. In our research (Hoffman et al., 1985),
we studied profoundly demented individuals who were able, with effort,
to raise their heads in response to our positive emotional messages
and look right at us. We felt the connection on a deep level, even
though these individuals could not speak.

Gesturing

A hand repeatedly slides across the surface of a table; a man's foot
taps over and over on the rest of his wheelchair; a resident strokes
her chin as you talk with her. You may see individuals making these
and other such gestures, but what do they mean?

When gestures are used, they can give added information about a
message or feeling, particularly with regard to the intensity of the
emotion (Argyle, 1988). However, gestures are difficult to interpret.
There are three factors that may contribute to this difficulty: the
gestures may be fairly complex, they may be subtle, or they may happen
quite rapidly, before you have a chance to process the information
(Emmert & Donaghy, 1981).

However, because a stroke, arthritis, or other age-related changes
may make movement more difficult, it is likely that gestures made by
many residents will not happen very quickly, they will probably not
be subtle, and they may not be complex. In fact, a single gesture may
be acted out over and over when the resident is unable to stop repeating
a particular behavior. This could make interpretation of residents'
gestures somewhat easier.

Posture

Interpreting a nonverbal message from a resident's posture may be
difficult if he or she is in a gerichair or wheelchair, perhaps somewhat

slumped over because of contractures or a lack of muscle tone. However, it is possible to get an idea about a person's feelings about the situation. Bartol (1979) suggests that observing a person's posture, among other nonverbal signals, is very helpful in understanding nonreceptive behavior.

> If the patient backs away from you, turns his head or body away, walks away, avoids eye contact, pulls away from you, shrinks away from being touched, tells you to go away, frowns, increases general body muscle tension, narrows eyes, closes eyes, or increases any overt sign of anxiety, the patient is nonreceptive. (Bartol, 1979)

If one ignores these cues and continues to interact with the person, there may be a catastrophic reaction.

The resident's posture can also tell you about his or her general emotional state. If he or she is walking more slowly than usual, with hunched shoulders, he or she may be feeling hopeless or depressed. A key to understanding what postural changes may mean is to know the typical postures of the residents—how they usually sit, if they lean to one side, if they usually look down toward the ground. If you have a sense of the normal posture, then any change, however slight, may be assessed. Because elderly residents may be considerably constricted in their movements, even a slight change may carry an important message.

Of course, increased restlessness is very important to observe. If some residents have increased their pacing, are jiggling feet, or rubbing body parts, you might suspect they possibly have to use the bathroom, have an infection, or are feeling anxious or upset.

Vocalizations

Even when you can't make sense of a person's words or their attempts to speak, you can listen for clues in the speed, pitch, and volume used in vocalizing. When someone speaks in a loud tone of voice, it is more likely to arouse concern than if the person speaks more quietly. When a resident speaks at an excessive rate, this indicates that the person may be losing self-control or feeling anxious, and is less able to cope with the demands of the situation. When this happens, it might be a good idea to wait until the person is feeling calmer before approaching again.

PROBLEMS IN INTERPRETING NONVERBAL MESSAGES

Have you ever told anyone, "I feel fine," when you really felt terrible? Sometimes people say the opposite of how they actually feel because they don't want to bother or worry anyone, or because they don't know how others will react to their true feelings.

Mr. James would grimace as if he were in pain, leaning over in his chair and moaning. When the nurse asked if something was wrong, he insisted, "I'm all right; I'm all right." Mr. James may be denying anything is wrong because he doesn't want to "make waves."

Not only do people hide their emotions with their verbal responses, but they may try to cover up a negative, nonverbal reaction with a more acceptable, positive one. For example, if a resident's blood pressure has to be taken, but he or she hates the feeling of the cuff, he or she may cover up an initial flash of anger with a smile or laugh. Residents realize that they may not have much power or control in relation to their caregivers, and they often do not want to do something that may alienate staff and affect the quality of caregiving.

AIDS TO INTERPRETING RESIDENTS' NONVERBAL MESSAGES

Information has been provided about how to be more aware of an individual's eyes, facial expressions, gestures, posture, and vocalizations as a way to understand his or her emotions and needs. In most cases, this is not enough. We often must have more information before we can understand the content and urgency of a message. There are several other strategies that can be used to increase our understanding: using feeling identification to determine residents' emotions, asking questions in a simplified, direct manner, and considering the context of the situation.

Feeling Identification

By observing facial expressions, watching for gestures and posture, and listening for voice tone, caregivers may have a pretty good idea of what residents are feeling, but may not be quite sure they are right. This is an excellent opportunity for using the communication technique of feeling identification (Danish & Hauer, 1977). With this technique residents are told a suggestion about how they might be feeling.

For example, a resident is sitting in front of the television in a room. A caregiver goes in and wheels the resident out to a physical-therapy appointment. The resident starts yelling and banging on the arms of the chair. The caregiver says, "It seems like you are angry about being taken away from your room." If correct, the resident might become more relaxed, calmer, less upset.

When people lose the ability to communicate as effectively as they once could, it can be a very scary feeling, leading them to wonder if their needs will be met. It can be quite frustrating and discouraging to be misunderstood. With feeling identification, knowing that someone understands can bring a welcome sense of calm and relief.

This technique should not be avoided because the initial feeling identified may be wrong. If the caregiver guesses angry when the resident is actually sad, residents may try to correct the caregiver or just shake their heads, in which case the caregiver could suggest a different emotion. At least by trying, the caregiver shows concern and caring, as well as interest in the residents as human beings.

The following is a list of some of the feelings that elderly residents may be experiencing (Danish & Hauer, 1977):

anger	despair	defensiveness
wrath	resentment	amusement
indignation	boredom	affection
happiness	pain	worry
joy	frustration	surprise
sadness	confusion	fear
loneliness	sympathy	disbelief
contentment	disgust	disappointment
love	irritation	

By pointing out some of these emotions to residents, they are helped to feel understood and comforted. We all benefit from having others acknowledge and share our pain and joy.

Questioning

Questions may provide new information if they are asked in such a way that the resident has a clear-cut choice, making them simple to answer. "Would you like me to turn off your light?" is a simple, direct question that gives residents a yes/no choice. When they respond, it will be clear just what they want. A less effective way of asking about the same situation would be: "You don't think it is too bright in here, do you?" This is confusing and perhaps puts pressure on the resident.

By asking yes/no type questions, even residents who can no longer speak can make their needs known by nodding or shaking their head in response to questions. Although open-ended questions (questions that begin with who, what, where, when, why, and how) can elicit more information, they may be difficult for the dementia resident to answer.

Considering the Context and Background

A third way of enhancing understanding of a resident's feelings is to consider the context of the situation. Factors to think about: What time of day is it? What other people are around? Is there a change in the routine of the resident?

The situational environment is not the only contributing factor to resident behavior problems. Residents' long-term memories can affect how they perceive what is going on around them. Knowing personal histories can help caregivers understand residents' feelings and actions.

> *Mr. Brown did not recognize the stout, gray-haired, elderly visitor as his wife, who had been slim and blond in her youth. He accused his visitor of being a stranger who had no right to be hugging him.*

You may also have a resident who remembers and feels proud of an earlier profession as a medical doctor or college professor. This person may react with more alertness when called "Dr. Smith" than when called "Pops."

Knowing the resident's normal routine is quite important for understanding difficult behavior.

Mrs. Lawrence was very upset one morning as the aides were getting her up for the day. They were brushing her hair, and she was visibly agitated, yelling and shaking her head back and forth, trying to push them away with her hands. When the head nurse came in and saw this, she realized what was upsetting Mrs. Lawrence. The resident had always taken great pride in being neat and clean. She would look in her hand mirror and smooth her hair into place with her hands. On this particular morning, however, her mirror could not be found, so she had no way of checking her appearance. This worried and upset her, and she let the staff know of her displeasure nonverbally.

This is an example of how you can use an understanding of the situation and background to determine what might be bothering or pleasing the resident.

WHEN USING VERBAL COMMUNICATION

Of course, interactions with residents are verbal as well as nonverbal. They involve a great many instructions, explanations, directions, and questions. Before speaking to a resident, it is helpful to identify oneself each time and not to expect the resident to remember one person consistently. It is important to use clear, concrete, familiar language with dementia residents. Convey only one idea at a time, speaking simply and not too fast. Try not to use jargon, although that is difficult for us in medical or nursing settings. The word "benign" can sound very ominous to a dementia resident. The speaker should use short sentences, and if the resident does not understand, repeat exactly what was just said. This allows time for the resident's brain to process the information. If the words are varied, this requires a greater effort for the resident. If the listener still cannot understand, the same thing can be said in a different way, perhaps using other words that the resident may remember. Of course, the verbal language should be accompanied by many gestures. When residents do try to answer and lose their train of thought, the caregiver might repeat back their last few words as a reminder.

Caregivers are often tempted to give lengthy explanations as to why they are doing something, or why the resident should be acting differently. Dementia residents, however, may not understand these explanations. It is far better to be sympathetic and understanding and address, instead, the underlying fears or concerns of the resident.

When Mrs. White walks into another resident's room, she might not understand you when you say, "This is not your room. You have no business being in here. Residents should not wander into the rooms of other residents." She will understand your empathy, however, if you remark, "I see you are lost. Let's go back to your own room" as you walk her down the hall. Even if she can't understand these words, she will pick up on the understanding and helpfulness.

In addition to being direct and concrete, the speaker should also use nouns instead of pronouns. The dementia resident loses track of who the pronouns are referring to. Therefore, the name or noun should simply be repeated again. Don't say, "Your husband is coming to visit; do you want to go to the birthday party with *him*?" Instead, repeat the noun over again by saying, "Do you want to go to the birthday party with *your husband*?"

Dementia residents often can't understand the commonly used contraction "don't." It is better to rephrase instructions positively. Instead of remarking, "Don't sit outside, as it is too cold out," one should say, "Sit in the dayroom today."

If dementia residents can't understand spoken language, written communication might be helpful. However, toward the middle stages of Alzheimer's disease, a demented person can read words but not understand their meaning. Therefore, if residents read signs, newspapers, or books, they are not necessarily processing the information. They may from habit be flipping the pages, perhaps noticing the pictures. The routine may be comforting, such as reading a morning newspaper. But the meaning of the words is no longer understood. To test whether the resident can understand written communication, a command should be written out such as "CLOSE YOUR EYES" so that the resident can read and follow it. If the resident cannot perform what is written, it is clear that written words are no longer meaningful to the resident.

Although dementia residents may have difficulty understanding language, at times they may understand. It is wisest for caregivers to assume that the residents can understand; this will keep caregivers from talking in front of residents and perhaps upsetting them with their comments.

TAKING TIME WITH DEMENTIA RESIDENTS

Elderly residents are sending out many messages through their facial expressions, gestures, posture, and vocalizations. Caregivers can observe these nonverbal behaviors and supplement this information by using feeling identification, asking questions effectively, and considering the context of the situation. Although it may not be possible to interpret nonverbal messages all the time with 100% accuracy, the effort has beneficial effects for both the caregiver and residents. The residents may be calmer because of the attempts to understand them, and in understanding them better, caregivers may feel less frustrated as well. Taking time may reward caregivers with happier, less annoying, or less difficult residents. A few minutes spent listening with undivided attention, instead of simply keeping an ear open while making a bed or giving a bath, can reassure residents that they are worthwhile human beings. They may become less demanding over time simply because the caregiver took the time to establish a trusting, caring relationship.

When residents are very demented, it may be difficult to treat them as responsive human beings. Caregivers are often very tempted to talk about them as if they were not there. They may forget to talk directly to them, especially if they never expect to get an answer in return. This can create a cycle of increasing withdrawal and passivity in the resident. We want to recommend that the caregiver simply try a bit harder to communicate with demented residents, remembering especially to use nonverbal elements of communication—voice tone, touch, facial expression, gestures, and use of personal space. Also, it is helpful to show dramatically that one cares. If a caregiver truly likes and enjoys a resident, smiles should be exaggerated and hugs or a warm handshake should be given. All human beings need affection and attention. For someone in a nursing home, the caregiver may be the only person who can provide for these basic needs. So attention and praise should be lavished, and the caregiver may be pleasantly surprised at the result.

SUMMARY

The importance of nonverbal communication techniques is stressed in this chapter. Strategies for using nonverbal communication in a planned way are reviewed, and techniques for more effectively assessing residents' nonverbal messages are covered. Instructions for using clear, simple verbal communications are also given. Outcomes of applying these techniques include the development of a closer relationship with residents, fewer catastrophic reactions, and less frustration on the part of both resident and staff.

LEARNING EXERCISES

For these two-person play exercises, a partner is needed.

1. Hold your partner's hand in an Indian handshake, while asking the partner how it feels and about his/her plans for after work. Switch roles. Discuss the impact of this kind of touching.
2. Stand to the side of your seated partner. Rub your partner's back with one hand while discussing what the partner will be having for dinner. Switch roles but without the backrub. Discuss the impact of this kind of touching.
3. Imagine you are a caregiver, feeling disgust and anger at a resident's recent verbal and attempted physical assault against you. Say to your partner, the resident, "You know I still like you very much." Have your partner determine whether you mean it, and how the partner knows.
4. One of you plays the role of a resident with an expressive aphasia. You are extremely thirsty and want a glass of water, but you keep repeating "cake" when you mean water. The other partner should practice using nonverbal communication in an attempt to understand you—especially using gestures and facial expression.
5. Imagine you are a visitor to Mars. After an elaborate dinner, your Martian host shows you to a room and tells you to step into a swirling mass of smoke, of all the colors of the rainbow. How would you feel? What could convince you to step in?
6. Have partners "pour out their hearts," telling a true or invented story with a lot of underlying emotion. The other partner should use the technique of feeling identification. Switch roles. An observer should point out whether you used this technique correctly.
7. Have a volunteer stand before the class and convey different emotions (angry, sad, disgusted, and happy) while saying the

sentence, "I have some news for you." The group members should try to identify which emotion the actor is conveying and how they knew it.

POSTTEST

Place a "T" before true statements, an "F" before false statements, and a question mark before those you don't know.

_____ 1. A resident with senile dementia will often know when staff are in a bad mood.

_____ 2. It is possible to hide your true feelings by controlling facial expressions completely.

_____ 3. It is best to approach a resident from the rear.

_____ 4. Caretaker speech should be used with all residents.

_____ 5. When you stand very close to residents, they may feel uncomfortable.

_____ 6. If a resident is angry and upset, the voice tone should be high-pitched and one should talk very quickly.

_____ 7. The most effective type of question to ask dementia residents is one that is simple, direct, and can be answered "yes" or "no."

_____ 8. Residents who can no longer speak have no way of telling staff what they want or need.

_____ 9. Although dementia residents may have flat affect, they can still express their inner emotions.

_____ 10. If we are sending out positive, nonverbal messages when listening to residents, they will feel more secure and trusting.

REFERENCES

Argyle, M. (1988). *Bodily communication* (2nd ed.). London: Methuen.

Bartol, M. A. (1979). Nonverbal communication in patients with Alzheimer's disease. *Journal of Gerontological Nursing, 5,* 21–31.

Answers: 1-T, 2-F, 3-F, 4-F, 5-T, 6-F, 7-T, 8-F, 9-T, 10-T.

Blondis, M. N., & Jackson, B. E. (1982). *Nonverbal communication with patients: Back to the human touch* (2nd ed.). New York: John Wiley & Sons.

Budd, R., & Ruben, B. (1972). *Approach to human communication.* Rochelle Park, NY: Hayden Book Co.

Burnside, I. M. (1973). Touching is talking. *American Journal of Nursing, 73,* 2060–2063.

Danish, S. J., & Hauer, A. L. (1977). *Helping skills: A basic training program.* New York: Human Sciences Press.

DeWever, M. K. (1977). Nursing home patients' perception of nurses' affective touching. *Journal of Psychology, 96,* 163–171.

Ekman, P. (1982). *Emotion in the human face* (2nd ed.). Cambridge: Cambridge University Press.

Ekman, P. (1985). *Telling lies.* New York: Norton.

Ekman, P., & Friesen, N. (1969). The repertoire of nonverbal behavior. *Semiotica, 1,* 49–98.

Emmert, P., & Donaghy, W. (1981). *Human communication.* Reading, MA: Addison-Wesley.

Fast, J. (1970). *Body language.* New York: M. Evans.

Fozard, J. L., Wolff, E., Bell, B., McFarland, R. A., & Podolsky, S. (1977). Visual perception and communication. In J. E. Birren & K. W. Schaie (Eds.), *Handbook of the psychology of aging* (pp. 497–528). New York: Van Nostrand and Reinhold.

Hall, E. T. (1966). *The hidden dimension.* Garden City, NY: Doubleday.

Hess, E. H., & Holt, J. M. (1960). Pupil size as related to interest value of visual stimuli. *Science, 132,* 349–350.

Hoffman, S. B., Platt, C. A., Barry, K. E., & Hamill, L. A. (1985). When language fails: Nonverbal communication abilities of the demented. In J. T. Hutton & A. D. Kenney (Eds.), *Senile dementia of the Alzheimer type* (pp. 49–64). New York: Alan R. Liss.

Howell, R. W., & Vetter, H. J. (1985). *Language in behavior* (2nd ed.). New York: Human Sciences Press.

Langland, R. M., & Panicucci, C. L. (1982). Effects of touch on communication with elderly confused clients. *Journal of Gerontological Nursing, 8,* 152–155.

McCorkle, R. (1974). Effects of touch on seriously ill patients. *Nursing Research, 23,* 125–132.

Mehrabian, A. (1971). *Silent messages.* Belmont, MA: Wadsworth.

Montagu, A. (1971). *Touching: The human significance of the skin.* New York: Columbia University Press.

Northouse, L. L., & Northouse, P. G. (1998). *Health communication strategies for health professionals.* Stamford, CT: Appleton & Lange.

Preston, T. (1973). When words fail. *American Journal of Nursing, 73,* 2064–2066.

Ruffner, M., & Burgoon, M. (1981). *Interpersonal communication.* New York: Holt, Rinehart, & Winston.

Weiss, S. (1988). Touch. In J. Fitzpatrick (Ed.), *Annual review of nursing research* (Vol. 6, pp. 3–27). New York: Springer Publishing Company.

PART II

DEMENTING ILLNESSES

Chapter 3

Alzheimer's Disease

LEARNING OBJECTIVES

- To describe screening tests and other assessments used to diagnose Alzheimer's disease (AD)
- To recognize the characteristic brain changes of AD
- To list the potential causes of AD
- To describe current treatment approaches
- To outline the stages of Alzheimer's disease
- To recognize the need to keep up-to-date in the field of Alzheimer's disease research

PRETEST

Place a "T" before true statements, an "F" before false statements, and a question mark before those you don't know.

_____ 1. About 50% of people over the age of 65 have Alzheimer's disease (AD).

_____ 2. Aluminum is a definite cause of AD.

_____ 3. There are several excellent diagnostic tests for AD.

_____ 4. Lecithin improves memory in the AD resident.

_____ 5. Neurofibrillary tangles are found in the brains of nondemented elders.

____ 6. AD residents may give an inaccurate history.

____ 7. AD residents often experience infections in the terminal stage.

____ 8. Average life expectancy after diagnosis of AD is 8–9 years.

____ 9. Although AD residents may read words, they might not understand them.

____ 10. Caregivers often feel a huge sense of burden when caring for an AD resident.

Alzheimer's disease (AD) is now the fourth or fifth leading cause of death in the United States. From a recent past of relative obscurity where it was rarely acknowledged or understood, the disease has been a household word since the mid-1980s (Jarvik & Winograd, 1988). It has provoked books and articles, support groups and fund-raising, and much anxiety and concern in normally aging older adults and their families. Some individuals with only age-associated memory impairment (AAMI), the minor forgetting of names, nouns, and appointments, have come into memory disorders clinics for assessment, absolutely convinced that they have Alzheimer's disease (ADRDA, 1987).

According to Hendrie (1998), an estimated 6%–10% of the U.S. population over age 65 has moderate to severe senile dementia, with AD comprising two-thirds of these cases. If mild cases are included, the prevalence doubles. Jorm et al. (1987) identify that 1% of those at age 60 and 30% to 45% of 85-year-olds are afflicted. Epidemiological studies examining this disease are difficult to carry out and have several methodological problems (Evans, 1996). One incidence study by Hebert and colleagues (1995) demonstrated that incidence of Alzheimer's disease is 14 times higher for the old-old (people 85 years and above) than for those between 65 and 69 years of age. Nursing homes residents demonstrate very high rates of dementia, from 46% to 78% of residents (Hendrie, 1998). Minority populations such as African Americans and Hispanics may be at even greater risk for AD (Tang et al., 1998).

People with Alzheimer's disease are living longer after diagnosis because of the excellent care they receive from family and staff caregivers. The average life expectancy of the person with AD is 8–9 years after diagnosis (Barclay et al., 1985; Walsh, Welch, & Larson, 1990).

Answers: 1-F, 2-F, 3-F, 4-F, 5-T, 6-T, 7-T, 8-T, 9-T, 10-T.

DIAGNOSING ALZHEIMER'S DISEASE

Alzheimer's disease is quite difficult to diagnose, especially in the early stages. Larson (1998) points out that people are diagnosed usually 2 to 4 years after symptoms first appear. In the early stages the disease can present very differently in different persons. Some will experience memory loss and will get lost, some will withdraw from social events and activities, others will have severe personality changes, whereas still others might be having financial and judgment problems (Geriatric Panel Discussion, 1987). The DSM-IV criteria (American Psychiatric Association, 1994) include the following:

- memory impairment
- one or more problems in the areas of aphasia, apraxia, agnosia, or disturbance of executive function
- the above causing significant impairment in social or occupational functioning
- the above showing significant decline from the previous level of functioning not due to delirium or depression.

Aphasia means a problem with language. *Apraxia* is the inability to carry out planned motor activities, for example, picking up a spoon, even though the person can still do these things automatically. *Agnosia* is an inability to recognize objects, despite preserved sensory abilities. *Executive function* involves activities such as planning, organizing, or sequencing.

Given our current knowledge, the diagnosis is based on ruling out all other possible illnesses. Diseases and problems that look like AD include psychiatric problems (especially depression), acute infections affecting brain function, metabolic disorders, medication toxicity or polypharmacy, other chronic brain disorders such as vascular dementias, plus many other possible disorders. The physician and other health care team members must give a battery of laboratory, psychological, neuropsychological, brain-imaging tests, and a physical examination to rule out these other conditions. Such examinations are often carried out in a memory disorder clinic affiliated with a medical school or hospital. The person with suspected AD may also want to participate in a clinical trial of medication that is being evaluated. The medical examinations for this kind of study are usually extremely thorough.

History

A good history is important, but the physician should consult family members and caregivers whenever possible, as the individual may be inaccurate when reporting the history of the condition. Crystal (1988) suggests the following kinds of questions should be asked as part of the history:

1. When did the memory problem start—was it sudden or gradual?
2. Are there personality changes or unusual ways of behaving?
3. Are there problems with language? What kinds?
4. Has judgment been affected? Is the person taking safety risks?
5. Is the person depressed?
6. In what areas of activities of daily living (ADL) and instrumental ADL has the person deteriorated? Can the individual wash, dress, toilet, find his or her way, balance a checkbook, sleep through the night, work, participate in leisure activities, and so on?
7. Has the individual had a stroke, head trauma, or seizure?
8. What other illnesses does the person have?
9. Review all current medications. Has the individual had any unusual side effects recently?
10. Do any other relatives have memory or psychiatric problems?

Costa et al. (1996) suggest that a clinician should explore the following activities in which the person may have experienced increased difficulty:

- Learning and retaining new information
  Patient repeatedly questions; can't remember recent appointments, events, or conversations; loses objects often
- Doing complex tasks
  Patient has difficulty performing multistep tasks such as cooking or working on finances
- Reasoning ability
  Patient can't figure out how to solve work- or home-related problems such as a plumbing problem; won't respect social rules
- Spatial ability and orientation
  Patient has trouble driving, navigating, organizing objects at home

- Language
  Patient can't find the right words; has trouble following conversations
- Behavior
  Patient is passive, less responsive; more irritable than usual; more paranoid than usual; misinterprets visual/auditory stimuli

Screening Tests

Screening for AD is also useful, although a more thorough battery of neuropsychological tests is encouraged. In a popular screening exam known as the Mini-Mental State Exam (MMSE; Folstein, Folstein, & McHugh, 1975), several areas of cognitive functioning are assessed. These include orientation to date and place, short-term memory, attention and calculation, recall, naming, language tests, and copying a design. Examples of the items on this test are:

1. What is the year, season, month, date, day?
2. Spell "world" backwards.
3. Remember three objects and recall them after several minutes.
4. Read a sentence and do what it says.
5. Write a sentence.
6. What is this? (Individual must name two common objects.)
7. Draw two intersecting shapes.

Many aspects of brain function are assessed very quickly in this test, so it is not an in-depth examination. However, the entire test, which has a total score of 30 points for no performance errors, can give a rough idea of whether the individual is cognitively impaired in areas of functioning affected by AD. A score below 24 is indicative of dementia. The MMSE does not test for AD per se, only whether some kind of dementing process is going on. It is recommended that this screening exam be given every 6 months to assess any changes in function which are occurring in the individual. If the person gets worse, this is an indication that there is probably a progressive dementing disorder causing the change.

Another screening test for early Alzheimer's disease is the verbal fluency test (Bayles & Kaszniak, 1987). Very early on, Alzheimer's disease affects individuals' ability to think of names and nouns, as well as their ability to come up with different ideas. In this test, individuals must write down as many different words as they can think of that start with the letters F, A, and S. They are given 1 minute for each letter. AD residents come up with significantly shorter lists of words than do normal older adults.

Costa and colleagues (1996) highly recommend assessing functional activities as part of a dementia work-up. They suggest that a reliable informant be asked about the person's functional abilities using the Functional Activities Questionnaire (FAQ) developed by Pfeffer et al. (1982). The person's functional abilities are evaluated in 10 areas. Among these are paying bills, shopping alone, preparing a meal, traveling, understanding a book or TV show. This assessment instrument is included in Costa and colleagues' (1996) *Clinical Practice Guidelines.*

Paul Solomon and colleagues (1998) have developed a 7-minute neurocognitive screening battery. This battery includes four brief tests: enhanced cue recall, orientation to time, verbal fluency, and clock drawing. The tests are fairly easy to administer and sample a variety of cognitive functions affected by AD.

There is no special test or marker for Alzheimer's disease, although much research is currently devoted to finding one. Researchers are looking for special proteins or antibodies in the blood or cerebrospinal fluid, reactions to tropicamide eye drops, or unusual genes on certain chromosomes (Hoyne, Fallin, & Mullan, 1996). Genetic testing is available for early onset disease and in some laboratories for the E4 allele of apoliprotein E (APOE).

Krasuski and colleagues (1998) have found that shrinkage in the brain's medial temporal lobe, measured via MRI, could accurately predict 94% of people who later were diagnosed with AD. Brain-imaging tests are also used to rule out tumors, infarcts, and other lesions or problems in the brain.

To definitely test for AD, a brain autopsy must be performed. The pathologist is looking for the characteristic signs of AD, which are neurofibrillary tangles and senile plaques. These also appear in the brains of the normal aged, but in the brains of individuals with AD they occur in far greater quantities and more specific locations.

CHARACTERISTIC BRAIN CHANGES OF AD

The brain contains at least 10 billion nerve cells (neurons) and 10 times as many cells that support these cells, and each nerve cell connects with thousands of other nerve cells (U.S. Congress, 1987). In individuals with AD, cells die in key areas of the brain: the cerebral cortex (the outer gray matter of the brain), the hippocampus, and the nucleus basalis of Meynert. These are areas where nerve cells make or use the neurochemical acetylcholine to communicate with each other. Consequently, brain acetylcholine is greatly depleted in AD.

The brain is also divided into four lobes: the frontal lobe, the parietal lobe, the temporal lobe, and the occipital lobe. Each half or hemisphere of the brain has these four lobes. Although all lobes may be somewhat affected by AD, the temporal lobe is most disturbed. This lobe of the brain controls many important functions including language, memory, emotions, concentration, and sense of time and individuality (Gruetzner, 1988).

Two major structural changes that occur in the brain of AD patients are neurofibrillary tangles and senile plaques. Neurofibrillary tangles are twisted pairs of brain filaments. With AD, these twisted filaments are concentrated inside the neurons in the hippocampus and amygdala, parts deep in the brain that control memory and emotion. They also are concentrated in key areas of the cortex that help integrate information, affecting therefore the person's ability to make sense of information and decide what to do. Such tangles are also present in other dementing illnesses, and less extensively in normally aging older adults.

Senile plaques, found outside the neurons, are made of an abnormal lipoprotein called beta-amyloid, as well as some material from dead cells. Plaques in AD are mainly located in the cortex. The investigation of amyloid and APP (amyoid precursor protein) is one of the key areas for possible causes and treatments of AD.

Other brain changes include inflammatory activity in neuritic plaques, granulovacuolar degeneration, hyperphosphorylated tau protein, Hirano bodies, presenilins 1 and 2, and other changes (Cummings & Benson, 1992; Progress Report on Alzheimer's Disease, 1998).

Vascular damage in the white matter of the brain such as ministrokes and other atherosclerotic changes to blood vessels in the brain may increase the severity of the clinical symptoms of AD (Snowdon et al., 1997). These changes may look like UBOs (unidentified bright objects) on brain-imaging studies.

POSSIBLE CAUSES OF AD

One theory currently not in vogue is that Alzheimer's disease is really "accelerated aging." This theory states that everyone would get the symptoms of AD if we all lived long enough, but in certain people for some reason this happens at an earlier age (Ebly, Parhad, Hogan, & Fung, 1994).

A variety of theories of causation have been described (ADRDA, 1988; Bayles and Kaszniak, 1987; Glickstein, 1988; Jarvik & Winograd, 1988; Snowdon et al., 1997). Findings from The Nun Study (Snowdon et al., 1996) suggest that low linguistic ability (idea density in writing) in early life predicts AD in late life. Genetic predispositions to the disease are currently being investigated (Hoyne, Fallin, & Mullan, 1996; Progress Report on Alzheimer's Disease, 1998). If individuals have the APO E4 allele, they are at greater risk for AD. Some research- ers believe that AD might be caused by a slow-acting virus or other infectious agent or prion. Because Creutzfeldt-Jakob disease and kuru disease are caused by slow viruses, perhaps this is what also causes AD. Metals that are toxic to the brain, such as iron and aluminum, may be another possible cause. Brains of AD persons have been found to contain higher concentrations of aluminum. However, this might be a result of the disease rather than a cause, as workers in aluminum factories do not appear to have increased concentrations or higher rates of AD. Deterioration in the immune system, where the body attacks itself, is also under investigation. Repeated head injury also causes brain changes similar to those in AD. And the role of acetylcho- line reduction is a topic of great interest to researchers.

All these theories and the accompanying research trying to prove or disprove them have not as yet produced any definite cause for the disease. However, researchers are beginning to believe that AD may not be one disease, but many, or else a syndrome of many different causes (Hoyne, Fallin, & Mullan, 1996; Jarvik & Winograd, 1988). The ideas about various causes have also led to ideas about related treat- ments.

POSSIBLE TREATMENTS FOR ALZHEIMER'S DISEASE

One major focus of treatment has been nutritional supplements or drugs that assist in the production of acetylcholine or else prevent its breakdown in the brain. Because there is less acetylcholine in the brains of AD residents, and because this substance is needed for communication between brain cells, it was believed that supplementing the diet would help in the production of this substance. Lecithin, a food substance that is turned into choline, which in turn is used for the production of acetylcholine, was given to persons with AD in a great many studies. It achieved no significant improvement in cognitive functioning, however. Physostigmine is a drug that prevents the breakdown of acetylcholine in the brain. It has been given also with no consistent effect. Other approaches in animal research have included the transplant of cholinergic cells (Jarvik & Winograd, 1988). Katzman (1987) believes that nerve growth factor, which keeps neurons alive, may slow the death of brain cells in AD and therefore be a possible treatment in the future.

Various drug treatments and vitamin supplements are being developed to delay the disease or prevent its clinical presentation. Many herbal products are being promoted to enhance memory such as ginko biloba. The medication Aricept will slow the progress of the disease from 6–12 months for some individuals (Progress Report on Alzheimer's Disease, 1998). Estrogen, antiinflammatory medications, nerve growth factor, anti-oxidants, Vitamin E, folic acid, and other newer choline-enhancing drugs are still in clinical trials (Sunderland, 1998; Trehan, 1998).

For aging persons without any cognitive changes, it is important to use and challenge brain neurons, to maintain their vigor and continued branching. However, cognitive rehabilitation does not seem to work with moderate to advanced AD individuals and can, in fact, be depressing to their families, who begin to feel quite hopeless about the future. Classes in reality orientation are also ineffective, although it does help to orient the resident in a more informal way. Caregivers should introduce themselves every day and remind residents of their own names by saying their names as they provide care. Individuals with Alzheimer's disease lack the neurons and brain chemicals to learn new information. However, McEvoy and Patterson (1986) have found that AD individuals can, in fact, learn new motor skills. Dementia residents who were taught ADL skills repeatedly over a 4-month period were finally able to regain some of these abilities. Some even found their way to the bathroom on a regular basis. However, such training requires an ongoing daily commitment from staff, which is often not possible in busy institutional settings.

The current best treatment for AD is to make the individual as comfortable as possible, which includes managing behavioral problems, keeping the person healthy, and helping the person have adequate rest and appropriate levels of activity. Because Alzheimer's disease is a progressive and deteriorating disease, the caregiver needs to understand where the resident is in the course of the illness and then target interventions to this stage of the disease.

STAGES OF AD

Every person with AD will experience the disease in a unique way. However, there is a consistent pattern to the deterioration that lets AD individuals be classified into certain stages (Dooneief et al., 1996; Gwyther, 1985; Reisberg, Ferris, & de Leon, 1982).

Beginning Stage

The beginning stage of AD is a time of uncertainty for the individual and family. Is this the beginning of a brain disease? Even after being evaluated by a neurologist or memory disorders clinic, it is often too early to tell. Sometimes the family will know that something very wrong is going on, but they cannot get the individual to a physician to be assessed.

In this very early stage, which can last several years, the onset of the disease is unclear. The family cannot exactly pinpoint when the changes first began. The individual can look very healthy and is socially okay. Although some language problems are occurring, especially forgetting of names and nouns, the person can substitute words for those not recalled. Individuals with AD are quite good at covering up and confabulating (telling tall tales).

> The nurse asked Mrs. Anderson what she had eaten for breakfast that morning. Although she had eaten toast and coffee, Mrs. Anderson replied that she had had a substantial breakfast of pancakes and sausage.

On mental status tests, persons with early AD will also make up answers rather than protest that they don't know an answer. When subtracting 7 from 100, they will give a strange list of numbers, such as 92, 81,

70, 64, and so on. Depressed individuals are more likely to answer "I don't know."

AD individuals in early stages will get lost, forgetting their way home after years of driving the same route. Although they may do fine in a familiar setting because they can call on long-term memories about how to do and find things, they may decompensate markedly if they go on vacation or move. This situation often makes the family realize that something is very wrong with their loved one.

Mr. and Mrs. Brown went on a long-awaited trip to Greece. While there, Mr. Brown acted very strangely, and Mrs. Brown was afraid to let him out of her sight.

The person with early AD will take longer to carry out job tasks or household chores. Cooking will suffer, as the person loses the ability to carry out sequenced or complicated tasks. Bills will be ignored or else paid several times over. The individual may make lists for everything and write notes to jog memory.

The person loses memory for recent events.

Although Mrs. Evans is visited every day by her grandchildren, she often calls them on the phone and accuses them of never coming to see her. She often will forget appointments or go to them on the wrong day.

Of course, the person suffers a psychological reaction to these changes. The person may feel scared, out of control, depressed, anxious, and may cope by withdrawing, relying on routines, and avoiding going out or trying new things. The person may become very clinging and dependent on family. Some persons may try to deny these changes, and may become quite angry if family questions their judgment or tries to take over former tasks, such as driving a car. Paranoia is common as individuals with AD believe that people are talking about them or are taking their things away from them. They try to find outside explanations for strange things going on inside them, rather than believe that they are suffering from an incurable disease. And many people will become quite depressed.

Middle Stage

In this stage, which can last for many years, diagnosis is more clear-cut. Individuals must have constant supervision during this stage, as they are unable to manage on their own. Memory loss is even more profound than before, and judgment is significantly affected—the person may say or do anything. The AD resident will have more severe language changes with a loss of both speaking and understanding abilities. In this stage there is also some agnosia, a loss of recognition of familiar things, and apraxia, a loss of the ability to carry out intended actions. AD residents begin to have trouble recognizing family and friends. They will have lost the ability to concentrate and must give up familiar activities, such as reading or bridge. The same notes that once jogged memory will now not be understood. Residents will often perseverate, asking the same question over and over again or doing the same activity for hours. They may start wandering or pacing. Feeding, elimination, and sleep are affected. The person may begin to eat more or less—some individuals become very oral, perhaps comforted by food. Others forget to eat or claim they have eaten when actually they have not. Urinary incontinence may begin, followed by fecal incontinence. Because of apraxia, the individual may want to participate in ADLs but be unable to initiate an activity. However, if prompted or shown how to do something, the individual may be able to do it.

At this stage, behavior problems are quite common, as there is a loss of impulse control and normal ways of behaving. The person in this stage may show psychotic symptoms such as hallucinations and delusions. The resident may become quite hostile or violent. The agitation and aggression may escalate to the point that psychotropic medications are needed. Depression may also be present. Physicians will often prescribe antipsychotic medications, anticonvulsants, anxiolytic/sleep-inducing drugs, antidepressants, or some combination of these medications (Trehan, 1998).

Families in the middle stage often feel a sense of significant burden—they are losing the personality of the person they love as their duties and responsibilities for care multiply.

Terminal Stage

The final stage lasts for one to several years before death. Residents may be mute or have great difficulty speaking while some will moan or scream continuously. They may have difficulty eating and swallowing but want to put everything in their mouths. This hyperorality means that there are many safety risks in leaving out small items or poisonous substances. Terminal stage AD individuals may not be able to recognize themselves or any caregiver. Movement becomes uncoordinated, and contractures may occur. There is bowel and bladder incontinence. Seizures may occur. The person has an increased risk of bedsores, infections, and may die of an aspiration pneumonia. Although the losses in this stage are quite profound, caregivers sometimes find these residents easier to manage as they are no longer capable of severe behavior problems. The individual will be withdrawn and perhaps sleep a great deal of the time.

HOW TO COPE

Making sure of the diagnosis is the first place to start, as some dementias are reversible, although AD is not. The individual must be thoroughly evaluated. The medical community may also be able to refer caregivers to other support systems, educational activities, and helpful groups.

The Alzheimer's Association has chapters throughout the country. This organization funds research, provides education about dementing disorders, and offers ongoing support to concerned family members and caregivers. It is highly recommended that the Association be contacted as soon as a resident or loved one has a dementing disorder.

It is also important to be alert to new findings about Alzheimer's disease and other dementias. The National Institute on Aging and other organizations are funding research in both the causes and treatments of this disease, so new information is continually being reported. Many internet web sites are available with up to date information. The Alzheimer's Disease Education & Referral Center (ADEAR) provides free information, government publications, and searches. Their toll-free number is (800) 438-4380.

Be sure that the patient has a good primary care doctor. Once a diagnosis of dementia is made, physicians sometimes forget to look for and treat other diseases. Larson (1998) points out that in a group of 300 patients, the following diagnoses also affecting patients were overlooked: depression, Parkinson's disease, low folate level, arthritis, urinary tract infection, lung disease, heart problems, anemia, peptic ulcer, and other conditions.

Grossberg (1998) recommends that advance directives be discussed with the patient by the primary care physician while he or she is in the early stages of AD. Persons with mild AD can make competent and binding decisions about their future care. This protects all parties—the person, the family, and the health care system.

It is important to comfort the individual affected by AD. Often the individual with AD is extremely anxious and scared and may be having difficulty communicating this to the caregiver. Concern and caring are the current best treatment for Alzheimer's disease.

Caregivers also need to take care of themselves. They often tend to feel guilty about normal reactions to the unusual and inappropriate behaviors of AD residents. It is important to expect anything and everything. The AD resident will act in surprising and infuriating ways, and approaches that have worked in the past may no longer be effective as deterioration increases. This may make the caregiver feel frustrated, angry, at wit's end, or just burned out and depressed. The caregiver should get as much support and as much comfort as possible.

SUMMARY

This chapter reviews the specifics of Alzheimer's disease, its diagnosis, brain changes, causes, treatments, and stages. Diagnostic and screening tools are reviewed, highlighting those that can easily be used in long-term care settings. The senile plaques and neurofibrillary tangles that are present in Alzheimer's disease are discussed. The potential causes of AD are enumerated, including accelerated aging, slow viruses, aluminum, immune system changes, and genetics. Possible treatment approaches for the disease are assessed with recommendations for enhancing resident comfort. The main stages of the disease are illustrated, and coping strategies are suggested.

LEARNING EXERCISES

1. If you are a caregiver, identify five residents in your facility with a diagnosis of Alzheimer's disease. Decide at which stage in the illness is each of these residents.

2. Attend a meeting of the Alzheimer's Association in your area. Find out some strategies for handling the behavior problems of your family member or residents.
3. Call ADEAR at (800) 438-4380 and ask for the latest research reports on AD.

POSTTEST

Place a "T" before true statements, an "F" before false statements, and a question mark before those you don't know.

_____ 1. There is now a blood test that is used for the diagnosis of AD.
_____ 2. Neurofibrillary tangles and senile plaques are the two major signs of AD.
_____ 3. Acetylcholine is a dangerous substance to aging brains.
_____ 4. The occipital lobe of the brain is primarily affected in AD.
_____ 5. Amyloid is a substance found in the neurofibrillary tangles.
_____ 6. Individuals with Alzheimer's disease rarely lie.
_____ 7. AD comes on suddenly.
_____ 8. AD residents may want to put everything in their mouths.
_____ 9. It is most difficult to provide care during the terminal stage of AD.
_____ 10. The National Institute on Aging funds research in the cause and treatment of Alzheimer's disease.

REFERENCES

ADRDA. (1987). *Memory and aging.* Chicago: Alzheimer's Association.
ADRDA. (1988). *Directions in Alzheimer's disease research.* Chicago: Alzheimer's Association.
American Psychiatric Association. (1994). Delirium, dementia and amnestic and other cognitive disorders. In *Diagnostic and statistical manual of mental disorders* (4th ed., pp. 123–163). Washington, DC: American Psychiatric Association.

Answers: 1-F, 2-T, 3-F, 4-F, 5-F, 6-F, 7-F, 8-T, 9-F, 10-T.

Barclay, L. L., Zemcov, A., Blass, J. P., & Sansone, J. (1985). Survival in Alzheimer's disease and vascular dementias. *Neurology, 35*, 834–840.

Bayles, K. A., & Kaszniak, A. W. (1987). *Communication and cognition in normal aging and dementia.* Boston: Little, Brown.

Costa, P. T. Jr., Williams, T. F., Somerfield, M., et al. (1996). *Recognition and initial assessment of Alzheimer's disease and related dementias. Clinical Practice Guidelines No. 19* (AHCPR Publication No. 97-0702). Rockville, MD: U.S. Department of Health and Human Services, Public Health Service, Agency for Health Care Policy and Research.

Crystal, H. A. (1988). The diagnosis of Alzheimer's disease and other dementing disorders. In M. K. Aronson (Ed.), *Understanding Alzheimer's disease* (pp. 15–33). New York: Scribner's.

Cummings, J. L., & Benson, D. F. (1992). *Dementia: A clinical approach, 2nd. ed.* Boston: Buttersorth-Heinemann.

Dooneief, G., Marder, K., Tang, M., & Stern, Y. (1996). Clinical Dementia Rating Scale: Community-based validation of "profound" and "terminal" stages. *Neurology, 46*, 1746–1749.

Ebly, E. M., Parhad, I. M., Hogan, D. B., & Fung, T. S. Prevalence and types of dementia in the very old: Results from the Canadian Study of Health and Aging. *Neurology, 44*, 1593–1600.

Evans, D. A. (1996). The epidemiology of dementia and Alzheimer's disease: An evolving field. *Journal of the American Geriatrics Society, 44*, 1482–1483.

Folstein, M. F., Folstein, S. E., & McHugh, P. R. (1975). Mini-mental state: A practical method for grading the cognitive state of patients for the clinician. *Journal of Psychiatric Research, 12*, 189–198.

Geriatric Panel Discussion. (1987). Practical considerations in managing Alzheimer's disease. I. *Geriatrics, 42*, 78–98.

Glickstein, J. K. (1988). *Therapeutic interventions in Alzheimer's disease.* Rockville, MD: Aspen.

Grossberg, G. T. (1998). Advance directives, competency evaluation, and surrogate management in elderly patients. *American Journal of Geriatric Psychiatry, 6*(Suppl.), S79–S84.

Gruetzner, H. (1988). *Alzheimer's: A caregiver's guide and sourcebook.* New York: Wiley.

Gwyther, L. P. (1985). *Care of Alzheimer's patients: A manual for nursing home staff.* Chicago: American Health Care Association and ADRDA.

Hendrie, H. C. (1998). Epidemiology of dementia and Alzheimer's disease. *American Journal of Geriatric Psychiatry, 6*(Suppl.), S3–S18.

Hoyne, J. B., Fallin, D., & Mullan, M. J. (1996). Research update in dementia. In S. B. Hoffman & M. Kaplan (Eds.), *Special care programs for people with dementia* (pp. 159–179). Baltimore: Health Professions Press.

Jarvik, L. F., & Winograd, C. H. (Eds.). (1988). *Treatments for the Alzheimer's patient: The long haul.* New York: Springer Publishing Co.

Jorm, A. F., Korten, A. E., & Henderson, A. A. (1987). The prevalence of dementia: A quantitative integration of the literature. *Acta Psychiatrica Scandinavica, 76,* 465–479.

Katzman, R. (1987). Alzheimer's disease: Advances and opportunities. *Journal of the American Geriatrics Society, 35,* 69–73.

Krasuski, J. S., Alexander, G. E., Horwitz, B., Daly, E. M., Murphy, D. G. M., Rapoport, S. I., & Schapiro, M. B. (1998). Volumes of medial temporal lobe structures in patients with Alzheimer's disease and mild cognitive impairment (and in healthy control). *Biological Psychiatry, 43,* 60–68.

Larson, E. B. (1998). Management of Alzheimer's disease in a primary care setting. *American Journal of Geriatric Psychiatry, 6*(Suppl.), S34–S40.

McEvoy, C., & Patterson, R. (1986). Behavioral treatment of deficit skills in dementia patients. *Gerontologist, 26,* 475–478.

Pfeffer, R. I., Kurosaki, T. T., Harrah, C. H., et al. (1982). Measurement of functional activities in older adults in the community. *Journal of Gerontology, 37,* 323–329.

Progress Report on Alzheimer's Disease. (1998). Silver Spring, MD: ADEAR, National Institute on Aging.

Reisberg, B., Ferris, S. H., & deLeon, M. J. (1982). The global deterioration scale for assessment of primary degenerative dementia. *American Journal of Psychiatry, 139,* 1136–1139.

Snowdon, D. A., Kemper, S. J., Mortimer, J. A., Greiner, L. H., Wekstein, D. R. & Markesbery, W. R. (1996). Linguistic ability in early life and cognitive function and Alzheimer's disease in late life. Findings from the Nun study. *Journal of the American Medical Association, 275*(7), 523–532.

Snowdon, D. A., Greiner, L. H., Mortimer, J. A., Riley, K. P., Greiner, P. A., & Markesbery, W. R. (1997). Brain infarction and the clinical expression of Alzheimer disease. The Nun Study. *Journal of the American Medical Association, 277*(10), 813–817.

Solomon, P. R., Hirschoff, A., Kelly, B., Relin, M., Brush, M., DeVeaux, R. D., & Pendlebury, W. W. (1998). A 7 minute neurocognitive screening battery highly sensitive to Alzheimer's Disease. *Archives of Neurology, 55,* 349–355.

Sunderland, T. (1998). Alzheimer's disease: Cholinergic therapy and beyond. *American Journal of Geriatric Psychiatry, 6*(Suppl.), S56–S63.

Tang, M.-X, Stern, Y., Marder, K., Bell, K., Gurland, B., Lantigua, R., Andrews, H., Feng, L., Tycko, B., & Mayeux, R. (1998). The APOE-E4 allelle and the risk of Alzheimer disease among African Americans, whites, and hispanics. *Journal of the American Medical Association, 279,* 751–755.

Trehan, R. (1998). Drug management. In M. Kaplan & S. B. Hoffman, *Behaviors in dementia: Best practices for successful management.* Baltimore: Health Professions Press.

U.S. Congress, Office of Technology Assessment. (1987). *Losing a million minds: Confronting the tragedy of Alzheimer's disease and other dementias.* Washington, DC: U.S. Government Printing Office.

Walsh, J., Welch, H., & Larson, E. (1990). Survival of outpatients with Alzheimer-type dementia. *Annals of Internal Medicine, 113,* 429–434.

Vascular Dementia

LEARNING OBJECTIVES

- To identify the kinds of vascular conditions that may lead to dementia
- To recognize what symptoms other than dementia are common in vascular conditions
- To understand how the course of the disease is likely to be different in vascular dementia from that of other brain diseases
- To recognize the behavioral symptoms that are more likely to be present in vascular dementia than in other dementias
- To explore some specific approaches in caring for individuals with vascular dementia

PRETEST

Place a "T" before true statements, an "F" before false statements, and a question mark before those you don't know.

_____ 1. Brain damage caused by strokes or heart disease can make it difficult for a person to control impulses and emotions.

_____ 2. Recent research shows that hardening of the arteries by itself is not a major cause of dementia in older people.

_____ 3. Multi-infarct dementia results from many little strokes in the brain.

_____ 4. It doesn't matter what causes dementia (vascular or AD); it always leads to the same problems and deficits.

_____ 5. People who have had heart attacks rarely have dementia.

_____ 6. A person who has had a stroke toward the front of the left side of the brain will often show a markedly depressed mood.

_____ 7. Damage to the white matter (subcortex) of the brain can cause symptoms of dementia such as forgetfulness and slowness.

_____ 8. Controlling high blood pressure does not help prevent multi-infarct dementia.

_____ 9. Persons with vascular dementia have a lower death rate than those with Alzheimer's disease.

_____ 10. Persons with vascular dementia can be moody and unpleasant to interact with at times.

Not long ago nearly all problems with memory and cognitive functioning experienced by older people were thought to be caused by "hardening of the arteries" (Barclay, 1993; Hansen, 1994). When Grandpa was getting forgetful, the family was usually told, "It's hardening of the arteries, and nothing can be done." It is true that atherosclerosis is a common problem in aging. Atherosclerosis is the buildup of a waxy substance on the inside of the arteries that stiffens or "hardens" them and makes them less efficient at carrying blood. This decreases blood flow, with its nutrients and oxygen, to vital areas. It was assumed that the common dementias of aging resulted from atherosclerotic changes in the arteries of the brain. It was an easy explanation for the progressive, relentless decline of intellectual function in some older adults.

In recent years research has taken a closer look into the causes of dementia and found that the picture is more complicated than just hardening of the arteries. Blessed, Tomlinson, and Roth (1968) studied the brains of demented persons after their deaths and found that in the majority of cases these brains were full of neurofibrillary tangles

Answers: 1-T, 2-T, 3-T, 4-F, 5-F, 6-T, 7-T, 8-F, 9-F, 10-T.

and senile plaques. These changes are characteristic of Alzheimer's disease, but are not related to atherosclerotic changes. They also discovered that the more demented the person had been in life, the more plaques and tangles were found in the brain on autopsy. The researchers noted that up to 50% of the dementias in their subjects were the result of Alzheimer's disease, which is a disease of nerve cells, not a disease of the arteries.

However, a significant proportion (8% to 30%) of the dementias in the elderly is the result of problems in the vascular system (Barclay, 1993; Wade & Hachinski, 1987). The prevalence and incidence of dementia resulting from vascular problems vary by the population being studied: that is, hospital based versus community based; clinical diagnosis versus diagnosis on autopsy (Barclay, 1993; Tatemichi, Sacktor, & Mayeux, 1994). For instance, an epidemiological study in Sweden found that of their sample of very old subjects (age 77 and older), vascular dementia accounted for 17.9% of those identified as having dementia (VonStrauss, Viitanen, DeRonchi, Winblad, & Fratiglioni, 1999). In a study of autopsies of persons who died with dementia in Switzerland, 35% were found to have vascular dementia and 36% showed mixed dementia (Gold et al., 1997).

Vascular dementia is caused by interruptions of the blood supply to large and small areas of the brain. The interruption may be caused by a clot blocking an artery thus preventing blood getting to a certain brain area. The interruption may be caused by a break in a blood vessel that leaks blood into brain tissue. The interruption may even be the result of insufficient blood getting to a specific area of the brain either because of changes in the walls of small arteries (through atherosclerosis, amyloidangiopathy, etc.), which prevents blood getting through (Hennerici, 1995; Hansen, 1994), or because of periods of interrupted blood flow or pressure as a result of a heart attack, for instance (Barclay, 1993).

Ultimately, atherosclerosis is often the cause of the damage, in that it is often a piece of debris from the plaque inside a hardened artery that breaks off and produces a clot and blockage. Likewise, a small artery may be so weakened by the atherosclerotic process that it bursts, causing a hemorrhage. But the problems in vascular dementia are not simply the result of overall poor circulation of blood to the brain. The problems result from damage done to a specific area of the brain because of an interruption of blood flow to that area. This damage may accumulate over time, causing progressive loss of intellectual function.

TYPES OF VASCULAR DISEASE

Research, especially research using modern imaging techniques such as CT scans, MRI, PET and SPECT scans, has led to a much clearer picture of the brain and how vascular problems affect brain functioning. This has led to much discussion and some controversy as to how to classify and what to call cognitive difficulties and other brain dysfunction perceived to arise from vascular problems within or outside the brain (Barclay, 1993; Davis, Mirra, & Alazraki, 1994; Gold et al., 1997; Hachinski, 1994; Hennerici, 1995). However, several distinct types of dementia can be traced to vascular causes. These types are distinguished by location in the brain, extent of the damage, and the source of the cause.

Multi-infarct Dementia

Multi-infarct dementia (MID) results from numerous small strokes or other interruptions to the blood flow that cause small areas of the brain to die, leaving behind what are essentially tiny holes in the brain. The individual will show different symptoms depending on where in the brain these little strokes occur. Usually a person with MID will have damage in several parts of the brain, including both the cortex (gray matter) and subcortex (white matter). The damage shows up in brain imaging tests as multiple abnormally light areas or holes. This is referred to as a "lacunar state," because "lacuna" is the Latin word for space or hole.

Stroke

A person who has had a stroke that damaged a large area of the brain usually has some symptoms of dementia (Barclay, 1993; Censori et al., 1996; Tomlinson, Blessed, & Roth, 1970; Wade & Hachinski, 1987). Also, a more limited stroke that affects an area of the brain critical to cognitive functioning will lead to symptoms of dementia. However, not everybody who has had a stroke shows significant signs of dementia. It depends on the location of the stroke, the extent of the damage to the brain, and the recovery of function following rehabilitation.

Cardiovascular Disease

Persons who have suffered heart attacks or who have cardiovascular disease often have cognitive impairment (Barclay, 1993; Barclay et al., 1988). In one study, 40% of the subjects being treated for severe heart disease were found to have significant multiple cognitive deficits, such as memory loss or coordination problems. Having cardiovascular disease predisposes a person to the risk of brain damage by depriving the brain of needed oxygen during the heart attack or by causing a person to have multiple small strokes. Barclay (1988) suggests that 20% to 35% of the dementias in the elderly may be accounted for by cardiovascular disease.

Some people with hypertension develop a slowly progressive dementia that includes seizures and stroke like events. CT and MRI scans show abnormalities in the cerebral white matter (Pantoni & Garcia, 1995). On autopsy extensive white matter atrophy is found in their brains. This may be referred to as Binswanger's disease (BD) or subcortical arteriosclerotic encephalopathy, and appears to be caused by impairment of the blood flow to this area of the brain (Barclay, 1993). This condition may be simply a form of subcortical MID (Barclay, 1993; Tatemichi et al., 1994).

Formerly, most individuals with dementia resulting from vascular causes were diagnosed as having multi-infarct dementia. The DSM-IV (APA, 1994), however, replaced the diagnosis of MID with vascular dementia, which is a more general and inclusive diagnosis.

HOW VASCULAR DEMENTIAS ARE DIFFERENT FROM OTHER DEMENTIAS

By definition, persons diagnosed as having dementia will have memory problems. They also will show other symptoms of cognitive failure, such as poor judgment, problems in orientation, spatial difficulties, problems with language, or personality changes. A set of these symptoms will be present regardless of the underlying cause of the dementia. However, dementia caused by vascular problems can be distinguished from other dementias both by the accompanying symptoms and the course of the disease.

People with vascular dementia have other symptoms of vascular disease as well. Hypertension is the most common problem. Also, they will have had a history of stroke, heart disease, or of transient ischemic attacks (TIAs), a temporary stroke-like syndrome that clears up in a few hours. Diabetes is another disease that is often present in persons with vascular dementia.

The cognitive impairment that results from vascular causes has some characteristics different from other dementias. Usually there will be a sudden onset of memory problems or cognitive changes. This level of impairment will remain steady for a while, may even show improvement, and then suddenly get much worse. This is referred to as a fluctuating and "stepwise course." This stepwise course is unlike that of Alzheimer's disease, in which memory and other cognitive problems develop slowly over a period of months or years. With AD, problems may not be recognized at first, but they get steadily, progressively worse. In vascular dementia, there are more sudden changes.

In addition to the sudden onset and stepwise course, vascular dementia has other behavioral characteristics that distinguish it from Alzheimer's disease. Many of these characteristics are related to damage in the frontal lobes of the brain. They include difficulties with sustaining attention, self-regulation, planning and fine-motor coordination (Almkvist, 1994; Cummings, 1994; Villardita, 1993). Symptoms such as depression, delusions, and nighttime confusion are also common in vascular dementia (Barclay, 1993; Cummings, 1994).

It often seems that when compared to individuals with AD, individuals with vascular dementia preserve more of their basic personality longer. Although research (e.g., Verhey, Ponds, Rozendaal, & Jolles, 1995) has not necessarily confirmed this observation, it is supported by clinical experience. Individuals with vascular dementia also seem to retain their ability to react emotionally for a longer period during their illness than do those who suffer from AD. Thus, they seem to retain more of their lifelong personality for a longer time and do not seem so totally changed to family and friends.

Depression is believed to be more common in vascular dementia than in other dementias. Again, this has not been universally supported by research studies (Verhey et al., 1995). Apathy or lack of volition is often present in vascular dementia. Apathy, along with the tearfulness that occurs as a result of emotional instability, may appear similar to depression in many residents with vascular dementia. Individuals with vascular dementia tend to have more vague physical complaints such as dizziness, unsteadiness, or headache.

Emotional lability or emotional incontinence refers to an inability to control emotions. Emotional lability is characterized by rapid, inappropriate, and spontaneous mood changes (Wade & Hachinski, 1987). The person may be cheerful and then quite suddenly become tearful. This mood change is not under the person's conscious control, just as physical incontinence can occur without the ability of the demented person to control it. The person with vascular dementia demonstrates more emotional lability than the person with AD.

The person with vascular dementia may show focal signs of brain damage, such as problems with vision, problems with swallowing, a small-stepped gait, or problems speaking (dysarthria), weakness in limbs, seizures, or disturbances in sensation. The problems with vision may include the loss of sight in half of the visual field, for example, toward the left or toward the right. In other words, a person may be unable to see in a particular direction without turning the head. Such problems are rare in AD individuals, occurring late in the course of the disease or not at all.

There are other differences in the typical symptoms of vascular dementia versus AD. The problems associated with AD are caused primarily by damage to the cortex or gray matter of the brain. This area of the brain controls "higher" intellectual functions, such as using words and language, arithmetic, performing complex learned tasks such as dressing, and orienting oneself. All these areas are usually affected in AD, but they are affected in a more limited way in vascular dementia. Only one or two of these symptoms may occur, because especially in MID, the brain damage is confined to more specific areas of the brain and is less generalized than in AD. If these symptoms do occur in MID, it means that small strokes have occurred in the cortex of the brain.

The dementia symptoms the person with vascular dementia is likely to show are caused by damage to the subcortical white matter of the brain. Sometimes these are the only dementia symptoms a person with vascular dementia will show. These symptoms include forgetfulness, a slowing down of thinking and movement, mood changes, impaired attention, and less control over thoughts and behavior (Barclay, 1993; Cummings, 1994; Katz, Alexander, & Mandell, 1987; Kwan et al., 1999).

As mentioned, the course of a vascular dementia is different from that of AD in that there tends to be a sudden onset, fluctuating course, and stepwise progression. This is related to the small strokes that can happen at any time to persons with risk factors for the disease. These strokes occur suddenly, may decrease function and then have some period of improvement, followed by more tiny strokes causing more brain damage.

IMPORTANCE OF A CORRECT DIAGNOSIS

It is important to differentiate between dementia related to vascular causes versus the dementia of Alzheimer's disease. In vascular dementia, we are able to provide treatment that will directly affect the underlying cause of the dementia. We can treat the hypertension, atherosclerosis, or heart conditions through medication or surgery. This can slow down or halt the progression of MID (Barclay, 1993). In fact, researchers have noticed a decline in the prevalence of MID and stroke. This has been attributed to the aggressive treatment of hypertension and an increased awareness in the general public of the importance of maintaining a normal blood pressure (Wade & Hachinski, 1987). As yet, we have no way to directly treat the cause or causes of Alzheimer's disease.

Despite being able to treat the underlying cause of MID, individuals with vascular dementia have a higher mortality rate than those with AD (Aevarsson, Svanborg, & Skoog, 1998; Barclay, 1993). It appears that the damage to the entire body caused by hypertension and atherosclerosis leads to a higher death rate for these individuals. On the other hand, individuals with AD often seem to be unusually healthy and physically fit, at least early in the disease. Of course, since atherosclerosis and hypertension are each so common in our population, and since AD is the most common cause of dementia, many of the demented elderly will suffer from both AD and vascular dementia. As mentioned previously, research studies of the autopsied brains of persons with dementia have shown up to 36% of dementia cases are the result of a combination of MID and AD (Gold et al., 1997). This is known as mixed dementia (MIX). In MIX the symptoms, course, and progression of the dementia will show a mixed picture, and the mortality rate is the same as that of vascular dementia (Barclay, 1993). In addition, having both problems causes a synergistic effect in terms of more serious impairment of cognitive function (Snowdon et al., 1997).

CARING FOR RESIDENTS WITH VASCULAR DEMENTIA

Medical Conditions

Persons with vascular dementia typically have physical illnesses, such as hypertension, atherosclerosis, kidney disease, diabetes, or seizure disorders. The dementia is just one symptom of the illness. Many people with vascular dementia will be taking medication for high blood pressure or heart problems. They may also be on special diets, such as a low-salt, low-fat, or a low-cholesterol diet. In caring for the resident with vascular dementia, the caregiver will need to be aware of medications and diet, and to make sure the person follows the diet during mealtime and snacks. The caregiver may have to take the resident's blood pressure and pulse more frequently than for other residents in order to monitor the effects of the medication and the progress of the disease. These individuals may also have paralysis or weakness as a result of brain damage. They may be clumsy about handling things or unsteady on their feet and prone to falls. Caregiving staff has to be alert to hazards in the environment that might cause difficulty. Residents may also have trouble swallowing and have a poor gag reflex. This can lead to choking, requiring intervention by the caregiver. In addition, the caregiver must be alert to any setbacks such as a new stroke or TIA, a seizure, or a heart problem.

Behavior Problems

Providing care to persons with vascular dementia is sometimes very difficult. A recent study showed that—especially at the early stages of the disease—family caregivers perceived a greater burden in caring for someone with vascular dementia than for someone with AD (Vetter et al., 1999).

Mrs. Leonard, age 82, had three strokes several years ago. The strokes had left her with mild weakness on the left side and a seizure disorder. She was forgetful and slow about doing things. She also had diabetes and chronic urinary tract infections and was often incontinent. But she was able to find her way around the nursing home and was fairly oriented. She had difficulty controlling her emotions and temper, and she was whiny and complaining most of the time. If staff did not please her the minute she asked for something, Mrs. Leonard would lose her temper and call them names. At times she would be particularly impatient, and she had been known to strike out at staff caring for her. Sometimes afterward she would apologize and say she didn't know why she acted like that. On one occasion when her behavior was particularly difficult, Mrs. Leonard was found to have an unusually high blood sugar level. Another time her seizure disorder medicine was at a toxic level. There seemed to be a connection between her physical state and her behavior. However, even when her physical condition was reasonably stable, Mrs. Leonard was demanding and complaining about not getting proper attention, and staff felt continually frustrated in ever being able to please her.

Part of the problem was that Mrs. Leonard seemed incapable of showing when she was happy or pleased. Even when she was talking about pleasant experiences, her voice was fretful. She rarely smiled and usually had a worried, discontented facial expression, even when doing something she liked. This lack of appropriate expressiveness was also due to her brain damage. Her strokes had apparently damaged parts of her brain that control emotional expression in the face and voice.

A person with damage to the right side of the brain may lose the ability to use or understand gestures and facial expressions (Robinson & Forrester, 1987). However, the person might still be able to understand and respond to voice tone or touch. It all depends on the location and extent of the brain damage.

This case illustrates some of the behavioral difficulties that occur in a person with vascular dementia. The person may show disinhibition—an inability to inhibit impulses. The disinhibited person will swear or strike out when angry, or she/he will openly seek sexual expression when sexually aroused. She or he may be unable to control other emotions and show an emotional instability or unpredictable irritability. She or he may switch from being relatively content to crying or being angry with little warning or provocation. She/he may be apathetic with poor motivation, and she/he may show slowness and unconcern because she/he is unable to pay sufficient attention to what is important (Katz, Alexander, & Mandell, 1987). If her/his ability to use gestures and expression in voice or face is impaired, it becomes more difficult to understand his or her nonverbal and verbal messages. It is tiring and unsatisfying to talk with someone like Mrs. Leonard who always sounds complaining and looks dissatisfied no matter what the topic of conversation.

Many persons who have vascular dementia, especially those who have damage towards the front of the brain's left hemisphere, will have significant depression and will need treatment with antidepressants (Robinson & Forrester, 1987). Persons with damage to the right hemisphere will often show an "indifference reaction," seeming to act as if nothing is really wrong with them or bothers them.

One 81-year-old man who was confined to a wheelchair with severe left-side paralysis following a stroke expressed a desire to get some exercise. He said he was going to take up running. When he was reminded of his disability, he dismissed it by saying, "Oh well, I'll start tomorrow."

Such comments make a person seem unconcerned or lacking insight, but they occur as a result of the damage to the brain.

CAREGIVER APPROACHES

In caring for a person with vascular dementia there are several things that are helpful to remember. These individuals are likely to have physical deficits due to damage to specific parts of the brain. They may be clumsy and unsteady on their feet. They may be very slow moving. They may show a weakness in one hand. Or there may be a problem with speech, either in expressing needs or understanding what is said.

To illustrate how caregivers can adjust their own behavior to help the resident with vascular dementia, consider a person with a visual deficit. As a result of a stroke, the person might have vision problems of a very specific kind, such as inability to perceive half the visual field. These people may see well what is in front of them or what is to the left, but unless their head or eyes are turned towards the right, they will not see anything to the right. Furthermore, they may not even remember that they cannot see to the right without turning and forget there are things they ought to be aware of on the right side. This kind of problem is known as neglect. Therefore, when someone approaches them from the right and then speaks to them, they may be quite startled that anybody is even there. They may even feel frightened and protect themselves by striking out. This can often be avoided by being aware of visual problems and neglect problems in these individuals. The caregiver can either approach them from their good side or get their attention while the caregiver is still quite a distance away. In this way the caregiver is less likely to startle these individuals by being right on top of them before they realize you are there.

It is helpful for caregivers of vascular dementia residents to keep in mind that much of their impulsive behavior, emotionality, apathy, or cranky depression is the result of damage to the brain. Perhaps because of the relatively greater preservation of personality, caregivers sometimes expect these individuals to have better control over their behavior. They seem to be almost the way they have always been—then they do or say something really hurtful or careless. What they have lost as a result of the brain damage is the ability to stop themselves from acting on impulse, to control emotions. It helps if the caregiver is able to take such outbursts or insults in a matter-of-fact way, recognizing that it is not really directed at the caregiver personally and that the caregiver does not have to take it personally. Even saying to the resident, "I'm sorry you feel that way, but I still like you" can be helpful. This will build up trust with the resident so that future caregiving situations will go more smoothly.

A third thing to keep in mind is that because the disease affects circulation throughout the body and the functioning of the heart, residents are at risk for sudden medical crises. Such crises could include a sudden cardiac problem, another stroke, or a seizure. The caregiver needs to be alert to these possibilities so that if they happen, appropriate intervention can be started.

SUMMARY

Many persons suffer dementia and behavior changes because of damage to the brain caused by major strokes, several smaller strokes (multi-infarcts), or cardiac problems. Most of these people will have had or continue to have high blood pressure and other problems in the cardiovascular or peripheral vascular system. The symptoms of this kind of dementia and its accompanying behavior problems are often somewhat different from those seen in AD or other dementing illnesses. This chapter describes some of these differences and suggests ways to manage individuals with vascular dementia.

LEARNING EXERCISES

1. Sit in a chair that has armrests, and have someone lightly tie your right arm to the arm of the chair (to simulate paralysis). Try to perform certain tasks using your left hand, such as buttoning your shirt, eating with a fork, washing your face, or writing a note. (If you are left-handed, have your left arm tied to the chair and try using your right hand.) Discuss your experience with the group. What was the most difficult task? What was easy to accomplish? What kinds of things would have been helpful to you in completing the tasks? How did depending on your nondominant hand make you feel?

2. With a partner, role play an interaction with a difficult resident, who is demanding and complaining and has poor impulse control. One person plays the resident being angry, insulting, etc. The other plays a caregiver remaining matter-of-fact and nonjudgmental. After five minutes, stop and discuss the experience, your feelings, what worked successfully, and what did not work. Switch roles and repeat.

3. If you are a caregiver, think of a person you know who has had a stroke or multi-infarct dementia. What are some of the behaviors and deficits in the functioning of this person that might be related to the brain damage? List approaches you can use and things you can do to help the person compensate for these problems.

POSTTEST

Place a "T" before true statements, an "F" before false statements, and a question mark before those you don't know.

---- 1. People who have had a major stroke rarely have dementia.

---- 2. The progress of vascular dementia can often be controlled if hypertension or heart disease is treated.

---- 3. Alzheimer's disease and vascular dementia never occur together.

---- 4. A person with vascular dementia has other symptoms of heart or circulation problems.

---- 5. Weakness or poor vision may result from strokes or multiple infarcts.

---- 6. A person with damage on the right side of the brain may lose the ability to use or understand gestures and facial expressions.

---- 7. When a demented person says something insulting to you, it is appropriate to take it personally.

---- 8. By the time people have dementia due to vascular disease, they will not usually have another stroke or heart attack.

---- 9. Controlling their emotions is easier for persons with vascular dementia than for other people.

---- 10. Vascular dementia can result from damage to both the gray and white matter of the brain, while Alzheimer's disease usually results from damage to gray matter alone.

REFERENCES

Aevarsson, O., Svanborg, A., & Skoog, I. (1998). Seven-year survival rate after age 85 years: Relation of Alzheimer disease and vascular disease. *Archives of Neurology, 55,* 1226–1232.

Almkvist, O. (1994). Neuropsychological deficits in vascular dementia in relation to Alzheimer's disease: Reviewing evidence for functional similarity or divergence. *Dementia, 5,* 203–209.

American Psychiatric Association. (1994). *Diagnostic and statistical manual of mental disorders* (4th ed.). Washington, DC: American Psychiatric Press.

Barclay, L. L. (1988). Differential diagnosis of dementing diseases. *Age, 11,* 19–22.

Barclay, L. L. (1993). Vascular dementia. In L. L. Barclay (Ed.), *Clinical geriatric neurology* (pp. 90–100). Philadelphia: Lea & Febiger.

Answers: 1-F, 2-T, 3-F, 4-T, 5-T, 6-T, 7-F, 8-F, 9-F, 10-T.

Barclay, L. L., Weiss, E. M., Mattis, S., Bond, O., & Blass, J. P. (1988). Unrecognized cognitive impairment in cardiac rehabilitation patients. *Journal of the American Geriatrics Society, 36,* 22–28.

Blessed, G., Tomlinson, B. E., & Roth, M. (1968). The association between quantitative measures of dementia and of senile change in the cerebral grey matter of elderly subjects. *British Journal of Psychiatry, 48,* 797–811.

Censori, B., Manara, O., Agostinis, C., Camerlingo, M., Casto, L., Galavotti, B., Partziguian, T., Servalli, M. C., Cesana, B., Belloni, G., & Mamoli, A. (1996). Dementia after first stroke. *Stroke, 27,* 1205–1210.

Cummings, J. L. (1994). Vascular subcortical dementia: Clinical aspects. *Dementia, 5,* 177–180.

Davis, P. C., Mirra, S. S., & Alazraki, N. (1994). The brain in older persons with and without dementia: Findings on MR, PET, and SPECT images. *American Journal of Roentgenology, 162,* 1267–1278.

Gold, G., Giannakopoulos, P., Montes-Paixao, Jr., C., Herrmann, F. R., Mulligan, R., Michel, J. P., & Bouras, C. (1997). Sensitivity and specificity of newly proposed clinical criteria for possible vascular dementia. *Neurology, 49,* 690–694.

Hachinski, V. (1994). Vascular dementia: A radical redefinition. *Dementia, 5,* 130–132.

Hansen, L. A. (1994). Pathology of other dementia. In R. D. Terry, R. Katzman, & K. L. Bick (Eds.), *Alzheimer disease* (pp. 167–177). New York: Raven Press.

Hennerici, M. (1995). Vascular dementia—A changing concept. *Arzneimittel-Forschung/Drug Research, 45,* 366–370.

Katz, D. I., Alexander, M. P., & Mandell, A. M. (1987). Dementia following strokes in the mesencephalon and diencephalon. *Archives of Neurology, 44,* 1127–1133.

Kwan, L. T., Reed, B. R., Eberling, J. L., Schuff, N., Tanabe, J., Norman, D., Weiner, M. W., & Jagust, W. J. (1999). Effects of subcortical cerebral infarction on cortical glucose metabolism and cognitive function. *Archives of Neurology, 56,* 809–814.

Pantoni, L., & Garcia, J. H. (1995). The significance of cerebral white matter abnormalities 100 years after Binswanger's report—a review. *Stroke, 26,* 1293–1301.

Robinson, R. G., & Forrester, A. W. (1987). Neuropsychiatric aspects of cerebrovascular disease. In R. E. Hales & S. Ydofsky (Eds.), *The American Psychiatric Press textbook of neuropsychiatry* (pp. 191–208). Washington, DC: American Psychiatric Press.

Snowdon, D. A., Greiner, L. H., Mortimer, J. A., Riley, K. P., Greiner, P. A., & Markesbery, W. R. (1997). Brain infarction and the clinical expression of Alzheimer's disease: The Nun Study. *Journal of the American Medical Association, 277,* 813–817.

Tatemichi, T. K., Sacktor, N., & Mayeux, R. (1994). Dementia associated with cerebrovascular disease, other degenerative diseases and metabolic disorders. In R. D. Terry, R. Katzman, & K. L. Bick (Eds.), *Alzheimer's disease* (pp. 123–166). New York: Raven Press.

Tomlinson, B. E., Blessed G., & Roth, M. (1970). Observations on the brains of demented old people. *Journal of Neurological Science, 11,* 205–242.

Verhey, F. R. J., Ponds, R. W. H. M., Rozendaal, N., & Jolles, J. (1995). Depression, insight, and personality changes in Alzheimer's disease and vascular dementia. *Journal of Geriatric Psychiatry and Neurology, 8,* 23–27.

Vetter, P. H., Krauss, S., Steiner, O., Kropp, P., Moller, W. D., Moises, H. W., & Koller, O. (1999). Vascular dementia versus dementia of the Alzheimer's type: Do they have differential effects on caregiver's burden. *Journal of Gerontology: Series B, Psychological Sciences & Social Sciences, 54B,* S93–S98.

Villardita, C. (1993). Alzheimer's disease compared with cerebrovascular dementia. Neuropsychological similarities and differences. *Acta Neurologica Scandinavica, 87,* 299–308.

Von Strauss, E., Viitanen, M., DeRonchi, D., Winblad, B., & Fratiglioni, L. (1999). Aging and the occurrence of dementia. Findings from a population based cohort with a large sample of nonogenarians. *Archives of Neurology, 56,* 587–592.

Wade, J. P. H., & Hachinski, V. C. (1987). Multi-infarct dementia. In B. Pitt (Ed.), *Dementia* (pp. 209–228). New York: Churchill Livingston.

MANAGEMENT ISSUES

Managing Depression

LEARNING OBJECTIVES

- To understand how common it is for nursing home residents to be depressed
- To note the differences between depression and dementia
- To understand that some residents can be depressed *and* demented
- To identify how depression can contribute to "excess disability" in demented residents
- To list the often-prescribed treatments for depression
- To use supportive techniques to help residents lighten their depression
- To encourage residents to participate in activities which they find pleasurable

PRETEST

Place a "T" before true statements, an "F" before false statements, and a question mark before those you don't know.

_____ 1. Depression is often the result of the many losses that elders experience.

_____ 2. The knowledge that you are experiencing dementia will frequently cause depression.

_____ 3. All nursing home residents are depressed.

_____ 4. Depression is quite simple to diagnose in an older resident.

_____ 5. Most older people will tell you if they are depressed.

_____ 6. Pseudodementia is a rare and unusual form of dementia caused by a virus.

_____ 7. The Geriatric Depression Scale was designed especially for the elderly.

_____ 8. Excess disability means the physical disability that residents often get at the end stage of the disease.

_____ 9. Depression is sometimes unrecognized by older adults and their physicians.

_____ 10. Polypharmacy is a useful approach to treating depression.

SYMPTOMS OF DEMENTIA

Imagine that you have been forgetting appointments lately. In fact, you forgot the date of your husband's 80th birthday. Imagine that your joints have been aching. You think you may not be able to afford your utility bills much longer on this big house. Your favorite daughter recently called to tell you she was getting a divorce. And your husband's cancer seems to be causing him more pain.

How have you been feeling? You can't seem to enjoy life any longer—things that once gave you pleasure have no meaning any more. In fact, you can't seem to get yourself out of the house. You've been having trouble sleeping— falling asleep may be okay, but you wake up several hours earlier than usual and just can't get back to sleep. And those early morning hours are the worst. All your troubles seem to go in circles around and around in you mind. In fact, you really can't seem to concentrate on finding a way out of your problems. Should you sell your home? You can't make a decision. Your husband has been after you to eat more, but it's been too much trouble to force yourself to eat. You also feel pretty down on yourself—you aren't worth too much to anyone, not since the children moved away and you retired. Death might be a welcome relief. You haven't told this to anyone else, but the thought of death does cross your mind as an end to your troubles.

These are the symptoms of a clinical depression: Depressed mood, loss of pleasure and interest in life, loss of energy, weight changes,

---

Answers: 1-T, 2-T, 3-F, 4-F, 5-F, 6-F, 7-T, 8-F, 9-T, 10-F.

sleep changes, inability to concentrate, feelings of worthlessness or guilt, slowing down or agitation, and thoughts of death (American Psychiatric Association, 1994). Sometimes an older adult may not feel depressed, but may have some or all of the other symptoms of depression. Anxiety is also a very common emotion in the depressed person. The individual may feel nervous, unable to sleep, and have physical symptoms of anxiety such as pounding heart, stomach distress, or sweaty palms. Late-life depression is often associated with a more chronic course than early or adult onset depression (Lebowitz et al., 1997).

Depression is the most common mental illness in the elderly. Often, depression is the result of the many losses that elders experience. In the scenario above, how many losses can you identify? There is the loss of thinking and remembering abilities, the loss of health, the potential loss of home because of inability to pay utility bills, the loss of a daughter's happiness, and the potential loss of a husband to cancer. Although older adults usually cope very well with a single loss, or a gradual loss, it is these multiple losses that can often send them into the spiral of depression. Although a person may grieve normally for the loss of a spouse, the loss of a spouse plus health plus home plus financial security can create a very deep depression.

DEPRESSION STATISTICS

Research studies show that about one third of nursing home residents are depressed (Blazer, 1982); other studies assert that among cognitively intact elderly people in long-term-care settings—20% of new admissions and 42% of longer term residents—suffer from either major depression or dysthymic disorder (Parmelee, Katz, & Lawton, 1989 as cited in Kaszniak, 1996). Estimates of subsyndromal depressions— levels of depressive symptoms associated with a higher risk for major depression, physical disability, medical illness, and increased use of health services—for medically ill elderly and nursing home residents have been reported as high as 50% (Lebowitz et al., 1997). Overall, the lifetime prevalence for major depression is 20% to 25% for women and 7% to 12% for men (American Psychiatric Association, 1994 as cited in Smith et al., 1997).

Reifler (1987) found that almost one third of the residents with dementia are also depressed, whether or not they are in a long-term-care facility. Depression is the most underdiagnosed psychiatric problem in dementia, the most common source of excess disability, and the most responsive to treatment (Lehninger, Ravindran, & Stewart, 1998). This depression is usually present in the early stage of the dementia, when individuals are most aware of the changes they are experiencing. They are aware of all that they will be losing and are frightened and anxious, as well as depressed. As the disease progresses people will often forget that they are no longer the people they once were, and so are less likely to be depressed. The progression of the disease is in this one way a blessing in disguise, as the increased forgetting can help the dementia resident feel somewhat better.

DEPRESSION OR DEMENTIA?

Sometimes it can be very difficult to tell if an older adult is depressed; current estimates of major depressive episodes range from 5% to 30% of AD patients and approximately 10% of AD patients meet the criteria for major depressive disorder (MDD) (Lyketsos et al., 1997). Younger adults will usually easily tell you that they feel depressed. However, older adults may believe that their sad, apathetic feelings are a normal part of growing old. In fact, depressive symptoms afflict between 17% and 87% of patients with Alzheimer's disease (Lyketsos et al., 1997). They don't realize they are depressed, or they may be embarrassed about being depressed. The mental changes that often accompany depression may be the most visible symptoms of the problem. Elders with depression often complain of memory loss and difficulty thinking or concentrating (Wells, 1979). If you ask them to tell you the date, for example, they are likely to say, "I can't remember." Very depressed elders are resistant during testing for mental functioning—they simply say, "I don't know. I don't want to do this." However, if you encourage them, they often know the right answer. These thinking and memory difficulties in a depressed person are sometimes called "pseudodementia" (Maxmen & Ward, 1995). "Pseudo" means false, so this is a false dementia. It is sometimes very difficult for a physician to tell the difference between a very depressed elder and a mildly demented elder; in fact, 10% to 33% of elderly people with major depressive disorder are misdiagnosed as having dementia (Maxmen & Ward, 1995). Although there is "considerable preliminary evidence for an association between depression and subsequent onset of dementia, especially when the depression occurs in elderly patients; is associated with reversible cognitive impairment; and has its first onset later in life" (van Reekum, Simard, Clarke, Binns, & Conn, 1999, p. 152); however, it should be noted that there are limitations to these findings and depression needs to be ruled out from dementia and vice versa. A depressed elder can receive a diagnosis of dementia. This is quite a serious error, as dementia has no current treatment, while depression can easily be treated and improved. However, it must first be realized that the individual is indeed depressed. To complicate matters, 15% to 20% of elderly with dementia also have a major depressive disorder (Maxment & Ward, 1995).

The Geriatric Depression Scale (Brink et al., 1982) was developed especially for a geriatric population. This instrument could be given to all residents on admission to a facility or to those residents who are thought to be depressed. It can be repeated every few months to track the level of depression in the residents and the effectiveness of the treatments they are receiving. In order to use this instrument, each question should be read out loud. The question may have to be repeated in order to get a response that is clearly a yes or no. The Geriatric Depression Scale loses validity as dementia increases.

EXCESS DISABILITY

A demented resident can also be depressed. In addition to the memory changes associated with dementia, the demented individual can have even more difficulty in thinking and remembering because of the depression. And the resident can also have the other symptoms of depression—withdrawal, lack of interest in life, feelings of worthlessness. These symptoms added on to the problems of dementia can cause "excess disability" (Kahn, 1977); two studies in elderly patients have found that residual depressive symptoms are associated longitudinally with significant disability (Steffens, Hays, & Krishnan, 1999, p. 39). In terms of depression, disability can include impairment in occupational functioning and problems with competence in self-care, provision of household needs, overall cognitive functioning, maintenance of role within the family structure, and extent and character of social interaction (Steffens, Hays, & Krishnan, 1999). Excess disability means that a person will experience more deterioration than is accounted for by the disease itself. If the disease causes behavior changes, the person will have much more behavior change than is normal for that stage of the illness. Excess disability from depression may cause the resident to cry more, to wander more, to be more disoriented than normal, to sleep less, to eat less or more, to moan or scream more, to refuse to participate in activities normally enjoyed, to resist care more, to be more helpless than is necessary, and so on; specific depressive symptomatology associated with disability include depressed mood, apathy, and suicidal ideation, anxiety, psychomotor retardation, and weight loss (Steffens et al., 1999). Clearly, it is very important for the depression to be treated, as the resident may improve markedly, even with a dementing disease. This does not mean that the demented disorder itself improves, but it does mean that the extra problems caused by other disorders can be helped. In addition to depression, other conditions may also cause excess disability—a physical illness that is not being treated, hearing and vision problems, being socially cut off, or being treated too much like a helpless child. It is very challenging to figure out what may be contributing to excess disability in nursing home residents. However, empirically validated research studies suggest that treatment for depression can reduce excessive levels of disability and result in improved levels of functioning (Lebowitz et al., 1997).

SUICIDAL BEHAVIOR

Very few individuals who complete suicide have been treated by mental health professionals (Caine, Lyness, & Conwell, 1996). Yet, in some research samples, 51% to 75% of the suicide completers over 50 years of age had seen their primary physicians within 1 month of death (Caine et al., 1996). In a small yet significant percentage of older adults, a profound depression can lead to suicide; "the elderly have been found to have one of the highest rates of suicide, involving primarily older White men, for whom suicide increase dramatically from age 65 to 85+" (National Center for Health Statistics, 1993 as cited in Kaszniak, 1996, p. 166). If not directly trying to commit suicide, depressed elders might indirectly try to kill themselves (Nelson & Farberow, 1980). This is called "indirect self-destructive behavior" (ISDB). ISDB may include such behaviors as not eating, having accidents, not complying with a medication regimen, leaving lit cigarettes around, and getting into fights. These kinds of behaviors may lead to a resident's death, which is the reason the depressed person is behaving in this way. Their emotions may be so overwhelming, so devastating, that they see no reason to go on living, yet they may be unable to directly kill themselves. Engaging in ISDB may ultimately lead to death. In some research samples 51% to 75% of the suicide completers over 50 years of age had seen their treating physicians within 1 month of death (Caine et al., 1996). However, suicidal attempts may be a cry for help, a way to call attention to the pain and suffering an individual is experiencing. A physician or mental health professional should be consulted for severe depression or suicidal behavior.

TREATMENTS FOR DEPRESSION

Often depression will not be treated in an elder. Why not? Sometimes the depression is not diagnosed. Older adults may not even realize they are depressed. Many older persons think the sadness, slowness, sleep and eating problems, and memory changes are simply normal changes of aging. Unfortunately, so do their physicians and caregivers (Olsen et al., 1988). Although some of the changes of depression may appear similar to normal aging, such as change in sleep patterns or a mild slowing down, the changes caused by depression are usually much more severe than the changes of normal aging.

Self-Treatment

People who do not see a physician for the symptoms caused by depression may sometimes try to treat themselves. They may take large doses of vitamins. They may ask for medicine from friends or else buy over-the-counter medications, perhaps sleeping medications, which may make the condition worse. Some adults try to "self-medicate" through excessive use of alcohol. Although the alcohol may in fact create some forgetting and blocking out of what is causing the emotional pain, it will cause many additional problems for the elder. Some adults try to control their depression through exercise, which is a more positive way in which to cope.

Medications

Medications are often prescribed by physicians to treat a severe depression; currently, there are multiple psychopharmacological interventions available. A class of antidepressants known as SSRIs (selective serotonin reuptake inhibitors) is now popularly prescribed (Hay, Rodriguez, & Franson, 1998). SSRIs may be more popular due to their ease of use, lower dosage adjustments, adverse-effect profiles, and greater acceptance (Lebowitz et al., 1997); Sertraline in particular is well tolerated by the elderly. This improved tolerability of SSRIs is based on lower incidence of anticholinergic effects, little or no influence on cognition at recommended doses, and fewer adverse cardiovascular effects (Schneider, 1996).

Other medications commonly prescribed for depression are TCAs (tricyclic antidepressants) (Schneider, 1996). These medications often take several weeks to begin to improve mood, so it is important for the older adult to continue to take the medication even though it may not seem to be working. Compliance with TCA medications is vital in maintaining consistent plasma levels; however, adherence can be difficult and needs to be continually monitored (Schneider, 1996). Tricyclic antidepressants can cause side effects, such as sleepiness, confusion, dry mouth, and orthostatic hypotension (a drop in blood pressure when getting up), or irregular heartbeat. Residents may need education about getting up slowly if they experience blood pressure changes when on this medication. And the side effect of confusion may add to the symptoms of the dementia. In fact, many elders who are on multiple drugs with these kinds of side effects may be misdiagnosed as having dementia, when they are really the victims of "polypharmacy"—being on far too many medications.

Electroconvulsive Therapy

For very severe depression, an elder may receive electroconvulsive therapy (ECT), also known as electroshock therapy. This is sometimes prescribed for depressed residents who have given up and refuse to get out of bed or even to eat, so that their very lives are threatened by the depression. ECT can be very effective—with reported response rates over 80%—and modern techniques for its administration are quite safe (Maxmen & Ward, 1995). ECT usually consists of six to eight treatments. Minor side effects consisting of short-term memory loss and confusion decrease significantly usually 2 weeks after the final treatment (Maxmen & Ward, 1995). ECT is often used with residents who have severe heart disease, who cannot tolerate the side effects of antidepressants, or who do not seem to benefit from such medications. The improvement with ECT is fairly quick and it does not cause any permanent brain damage or memory loss (Maxment & Ward, 1995).

Group Therapy

Group therapy can be helpful in increasing motivation, self-esteem, communication, and activity (Whanger, 1980). There are a variety of groups that can be carried out by nursing staff, activities staff, or a social worker or psychologist. The combination of group therapy techniques with the structured focus and time limitations of brief therapy offers the possibility for a wide distribution of therapeutic assistance to a variety of client populations (Garvin, 1990); some examples of group therapy techniques include remotivation groups, music therapy groups, recreational therapy groups, reminiscence programs, educational group activities, and other creative activities and events.

The opportunity to talk with other residents, to be stimulated by activities, and to be encouraged by a group leader will help a resident overcome depression. Residents should be invited to attend group activities but should not be forced to attend. Sometimes just watching the activity for several meetings eventually inspires the resident to join in. If the caregiver sincerely believes in the value of the activity and accompanies residents to the program, they will sometimes overcome their reluctance to attend. Depressed individuals usually withdraw and have little energy. They may want to go to an event but will find that they just cannot make themselves attend it. Encouragement is helpful. Depressed residents with dementia may prefer simpler activities, such as dance groups, music groups, exercise groups, or gardening groups.

Supportive Activities

It is very important to provide a supportive approach. This means supporting depressed residents by actively trying to understand them, talking with them and actively listening to them, discussing feelings, and giving real affection. Sometimes the resident who feels overwhelmed by losses can find comfort in simple substitutions, for example, a teddy bear to nurture, a candy bar that was once a favorite food.

A Sense of Control

Many residents are depressed because they no longer have a purpose in life, no reason to go on living. In a classic study, Ellen Langer and Judith Rodin (1976) found that by giving residents something to be responsible for, something to care about, the residents greatly improved their mental and physical health. The researchers gave two groups of nursing home residents a plant. In one group, the residents were told that the staff would care for the plant. In the other group, the residents were told that this was their plant to care for as they wished. Which group of residents improved? The group with responsibility and purpose, who had to care for their own plants. Such a simple intervention, yet with such profound consequences. How do caregivers take responsibility away from residents? Once residents are admitted to a facility, they no longer have control over even the simplest routines of their lives—when and what to eat, when to bathe, when to sleep, who their neighbors are. People who have to give up such control often feel very helpless, very stressed, and in much emotional pain. It is important for the caregiver to think of ways to give control back to the resident.

Cognitive Therapy

Cognitive therapy has been very successful in the treatment of depression (Beck et al., 1979); cognitive therapy is reported to be as effective as antidepressant medication in the treatment of depression with lower relapse rates than a pharmacological intervention alone (Moretti, Feldman, & Shaw, 1990). Gallagher and Thompson (1981) found that a program of increasing the number of pleasurable events in a depressed elder's life can help to decrease the depression. This is done through identifying those activities that a person finds rewarding and then encouraging the elder to participate. The elder also keeps track of mood daily and charts how mood is increased when participation in pleasurable activities is increased.

Pleasant Events

Caregivers need to discover what the residents find pleasurable. The Older Persons' Pleasant Events Schedule has been used to assess this (Gallagher & Thompson, 1981). Some of the activities on this instrument are very simple things, such as looking at clouds, receiving a compliment, listening to music, being with friends, reading a magazine. Yet they are what make life worth living. Caregivers need to help our residents experience some of their pleasurable activities, such as receiving a compliment. It is so easy to give a compliment—yet how often do caregivers rush through work so quickly that they don't notice when a resident has made a special effort to do something well?

Demented residents might change in what they consider pleasurable. Very often residents who used to love completing a difficult craft activity, such as knitting or crocheting, will find doing this same activity now can make them feel frustrated and worthless. Participating in the activity simply calls attention to their increasing problems with memory and coordination when they cannot complete the craft at the same level as before. In this case, it is better for the resident to do a simpler activity, like digging in a garden or listening to old songs. If residents cannot tell the caregiver whether they like a particular activity, the caregiver might question the family about hobbies or events they used to enjoy. Flatten, Wilhite, and Reyes-Watson (1988) suggest the following interest areas should be explored: crafts, sports, reading or writing, table games, music, intellectual activities (e.g., discussion groups, lectures), spectator appreciation (e.g., movies, sightseeing), clubs and organizations (e.g., church, civic groups), and other hobbies (e.g., photography, collecting things, bird watching, gardening).

Can providing pleasant activities really make a difference in the life of a resident?

Dr. Eugene Dagon (1988), a geropsychiatrist, tells the story of an elderly woman recently admitted to a nursing home. The woman seemed to adjust well. But then she began to act very strangely. She threw used pieces of toilet paper all over her room. Dr. Dagon interviewed her and found that she did not admit to feeling depressed, and she also seemed to be oriented to person, place, and time. However, the elderly resident's daughter had gotten sick herself and had not been able to visit her mother. And the resident's dietitian had put her on a diet, so that she couldn't eat her favorite chocolate candy any longer. One more thing, her sleep had been disrupted by another resident who screamed all night long. Dr. Dagon decided that his patient had experienced multiple losses, so he began to replace as many of her lost pleasures as possible. He had the daughter take the mother out for drives; he arranged for some diabetic chocolate candy; and he conducted a life review with his patient, having her look at old photographs and reminisce about the important people in her life. Within 3 days, his patient had improved remarkably and began to feel much better. On one outing with the daughter, an amazing thing happened. She met a retiring general who had liberated her from a concentration camp in her youth. This event was given newspaper coverage, and the patient received a lot of attention from the staff and residents of the facility. The patient was never depressed again.

All human beings find certain things pleasurable—favorite foods, a warm smile, a kind touch, attention, and praise. And then we each have certain activities that give us individual joy. Caregivers can make an effort to discover the unique pleasures of life for residents and try to provide them, as well as the universal supports that all of us treasure. Being acknowledged as a human being, receiving a warm welcome— these can be especially important to a demented resident. There is an unfortunate tendency to overlook these residents, to ignore their humanity, to talk around them rather than to them. However, some caregivers believe that dementia residents can take in much more than they are given credit for. In the rush and drain of routine caregiving, there is a temptation to pay less attention to the emotional needs of the dementia residents. They often can't talk with the caregivers. They may have less expressive faces. They do tend to withdraw sometimes. However, caregivers must be sensitive to the depression they may be experiencing and the excess disability it may be causing. Providing pleasure to dementia residents may be important treatment for alleviating their depression and can be as simple as a friendly hello or hug.

SUMMARY

Depression is a very common problem in elderly people. It occurs in people living at home and in those living in the long-term-care setting. The symptoms of depression can make a person appear demented. Also, persons with dementia can experience depression, causing them to seem more impaired than they actually are. It is important to be able to recognize the signs of depression in nursing home residents and to know what steps can be taken to help them overcome this condition. This chapter provides information about depression and its treatments. It also suggests approaches and activities that the caregiver can use to help the person who is depressed.

LEARNING EXERCISES

1. Think about the past year. Have you experienced any losses or traumatic changes in your life? What were they? How did they make you feel? How long did it take you to get back on an even keel? What kind of help, if any, did you receive to help you cope better? What kinds of things did you do to make yourself feel better—talk with friends, take up an exercise program, eat junk foods?
2. Mrs. Hawkins lost her husband 6 months ago, after 52 years of marriage. She had to sell her house, as she could no longer manage to keep it up on her own. She plans to move in with her daughter. Unfortunately, on moving day Mrs. Hawkins fell and broke her hip. On admission to a facility, she was put on a soft diet. Caregivers notice also that she rarely puts on her eyeglasses. Her daughter comes to visit very infrequently, although she does phone sometimes. Describe the losses Mrs. Hawkins has experienced. What can caregivers do to help her feel better?
3. If you are a caregiver, ask a resident or her family to list her most pleasant activities. Identify two activities you could help her participate in this week.
4. If you are a caregiver, pick out three residents who have moderate dementia. List symptoms of depression they might also be experiencing.

5. How can a caregiver give some control over their own lives back to residents? In what areas can residents make decisions for themselves?

POSTTEST

Place a "T" before true statements, an "F" before false statements, and a question mark before those you don't know.

___ 1. About one third of nursing home residents are depressed.
___ 2. Depression usually occurs late in the course of a dementing illness.
___ 3. Depressed residents are likely to say, "I don't know" when asked questions on a mental status test.
___ 4. Depressed residents are sometimes inaccurately diagnosed as being demented.
___ 5. A dementia resident with excess disability is functioning at an excessively poor level.
___ 6. Tricyclic antidepressants may cause additional confusion in a demented resident.
___ 7. A resident with orthostatic hypotension should get up very slowly.
___ 8. It is not possible for a depressed resident to participate in pleasurable activities.
___ 9. Sometimes dementia residents no longer find their past hobbies pleasurable.
___ 10. It is important to give compliments to depressed residents.

REFERENCES

American Psychiatric Association. (1994). *Diagnostic and statistical manual of mental disorders* (4th ed.). Washington, DC: American Psychiatric Press.
Beck, A., Rush, J., Shaw, B. F., & Emery, G. (1979). *Cognitive therapy of depression.* New York: Guilford Press.
Blazer, D. (1982). The epidemiology of late life depression. *Journal of the American Geriatrics Society, 30,* 587–592.

Answers: 1-T, 2-F, 3-T, 4-T, 5-T, 6-T, 7-T, 8-F, 9-T, 10-T.

Brink, T., et al. (1982). Screening tests for geriatric depression. *Clinical Gerontologist, 1*(1), 37–44.

Caine, E. D., Lyness, J. M., & Conwell, Y. (1996). Diagnosis of late-life depression: Preliminary studies in primary care settings. *American Journal of Geriatric Psychiatry, 4*(Suppl. 1), S45–S50.

Dagon, E. (1988). Managing depression in the nursing home. In P. Katz & E. Calkins (Eds.), *Principles and practice of nursing home care* (pp. 150–179). New York: Springer Publishing Co.

Flatten, K., Wilhite, B., & Reyes-Watson, E. (1988). *Recreation activities for the elderly.* New York: Springer Publishing Co.

Gallagher, D., & Thompson, L. W. (1981). *Depression in the elderly: A behavioral treatment manual.* Los Angeles: University of Southern California Press.

Garvin, C. D. (1990). Short-term group therapy. In R. A. Wells & V. J. Giannetti (Eds.), *Handbook of the brief psychotherapies* (pp. 513–536). New York: Plenum.

Hay, D. P., Rodriguez, M. M., & Franson, K. L. (1998). Treatment of depression in late life. *Clinics in Geriatric Medicine, 14*(1), 33–46.

Kahn, R. L. (1977). Excess disabilities. In S. H. Zarit (Ed.), *Readings in aging and death.* New York: Harper & Row.

Kaszniak, A. W. (1996). Techniques and instruments for assessment of the elderly. In S. H. Zarit & B. G. Knight (Eds.), *A guide to psychotherapy and aging: Effective clinical interventions in a life-stage context* (pp. 163–168). Washington, DC: American Psychological Association.

Langer, E., & Rodin, J. (1976). The effects of choice and enhanced personal responsibility for the aged: A field study in an institutional setting. *Journal of Personality and Social Psychology, 34*, 191–198.

Lebowitz, B. D., Pearson, J. L., Schneider, L. S., Reynolds, C. F., Alexopoulos, G. S., Bruce, M. L., Conwell, Y., Katz, I. R., Meyers, B. S., Morrison, M. F., Mossey, J., Niederehe, G., & Parmelee, P. (1997). Diagnosis and treatment of depression in late life. *Journal of the American Medical Association, 278*, 1186–1190.

Lehninger, F. W., Ravindran, V. L., & Stewart, J. T. (1998). Management strategies for problem behaviors in the patient with dementia. *Geriatrics, 53*, 55–56, 66–68, 71–75.

Lyketsos, C. G., Steele, C., Baker, L., Galik, E., Kopunek, S., Steinberg, M., & Warren, A. (1997). Major and minor depression in Alzheimer's disease: Prevalence and impact. *Journal of Neuropsychiatry and Clinical Neurosciences, 9*, 556–561.

Maxmen, J. S., & Ward, N. G. (1995). *Essential psychopathology and its treatment* (2nd ed.). New York: Norton.

Moretti, M. M., Feldman, L. A., & Shaw, B. F. (1990). Cognitive therapy: Current issues in theory and practice. In R. A. Wells & V. J. Giannetti (Eds.), *Handbook of the brief psychotherapies* (pp. 217–233). New York: Plenum.

Nelson, F., & Farberow, N. (1980). Indirect self-destructive behavior in the elderly nursing home patient. *Journal of Gerontology, 35,* 949–959.

Olsen, E. J., et al. (1988). Depression in the older patient: Common but complex. *Older Patient, 2*(2), 12–21.

Reifler, B. V. (1987). A strange, eventful history. In A. C. Kalicki (Ed.), *Confronting Alzheimer's disease* (pp. 1–10). Owings Mills, MD: National Health Publishing.

Schneider, L. S. (1996). Pharmacologic considerations in the treatment of late-life depression. *American Journal of Geriatric Psychiatry, 4*(Suppl. 1), S51–S65.

Smith, G. R., Mosley, C. L., & Booth, B. M. (1997). Measuring health care quality: Major depressive disorder. *Discussion Papers: Agency for Health Care Research.* Rockville, MD: Center for Quality Measurement and Improvement.

Steffens, D. C., Hays, J. C., & Krishnan, K. R. R. (1999). Disability in geriatric depression. *American Journal of Geriatric Psychiatry, 7*(1), 34–40.

van Reekum, R., Simard, M., Clarke, D., Binns, M. A., & Conn, D. (1999). Late-life depression as a possible predictor of dementia. *American Journal of Geriatric Psychiatry, 7,* 151–159.

Wells, C. E. (1979). Pseudodementia. *American Journal of Psychiatry, 136,* 895–900.

Whanger, A. D. (1980). Treatment within the institution. In E. W. Busse & D. G. Blazer (Eds.), *Handbook of geriatric psychiatry* (pp. 453–472). New York: Van Nostrand Reinhold.

Zeiss, A. M., & Steffen, A. (1996). Behavioral and cognitive-behavioral treatments: An overview of social learning. In S. H. Zarit & B. G. Knight (Eds.), *A guide to psychotherapy and aging: Effective clinical interventions in a life-stage context* (pp. 139–158). Washington, DC: American Psychological Association.

Chapter 6

Solving Difficult Behavior Problems

LEARNING OBJECTIVES

- To describe typical difficult problem behaviors
- To understand common reasons behind patient behavioral problems, such as a lifelong pattern of behavior, reactions to life stress, dementing illnesses, sundown syndrome or nighttime and sleep difficulties, barriers in the physical environment, or caregiver moods and actions
- To understand better the need for a caregiver to know the resident well and how the caregiver's behavior influences resident behavior
- To identify the use, effects, and side effects of psychoactive drugs
- To develop a treatment plan to solve difficult behavior problems using the principles of communication techniques

PRETEST

Place a "T" before true statements, an "F" before false statements, and a question mark before those you don't know.

_____ 1. Sundown syndrome is a term used to refer to people who are in the sundown years of their lives.

_____ 2. People who have lived alone all their lives easily adjust to life in a nursing home.

_____ 3. A person who is grieving may act hostile.

_____ 4. When persons with brain damage are in situations they can't handle, they may respond with a catastrophic reaction.

_____ 5. Residents don't notice anything different when staff are facing a crisis such as a facility inspection.

_____ 6. Shiny floors cause some residents problems because they see puddles on them.

_____ 7. Tranquilizers are often used in long-term-care settings to control problem behavior.

_____ 8. When a resident climbs into another resident's bed, this probably indicates interest in seeking out a sex partner.

_____ 9. Residents who ask repetitive questions do it to annoy staff on purpose.

_____ 10. Abusive dementia residents often can't control their behavior.

The day-to-day tasks of caring for residents in a long-term-care facility are often made more tiring, more trying, and more difficult by uncooperative, unpredictable, and even dangerous behavior on the part of the resident. Behavior problems in a long-term-care settings have been studied by several researchers (e.g., Allen-Burge, Stevens, & Burgio, 1999; Aronson, 1983; Burgio et al., 1988; Winger, Schirm, & Stewart, 1987; Zimmer, Watson, & Treat, 1984) and are exhibited in as many as 90% of persons with dementing illness (Davis, Buckwalter, & Burgio, 1997). In general, a very high incidence of problem behaviors has been found in long-term-care settings. For instance, Zimmer et al. (1984) found that only 35% of their sample of residents in nursing homes had no significant behavior problems. They found 42% had moderate behavior problems (showed impaired judgment and required physical restraint at times), and 23% of their sample had serious behavior problems (e.g., aggressive behavior, physical resistance to care, and uncontrolled wandering).

Winger et al. (1987) examined aggressive behavior in two Veterans Administration long-term-care settings. They found that 91% of the

---

Answers: 1-F, 2-F, 3-T, 4-T, 5-F, 6-T, 7-T, 8-F, 9-F, 10-T.

nursing home residents and 66% of the intermediate care residents demonstrated aggressive behavior. If behaviors considered merely disruptive were not included (e.g., shouting, cursing, acting impatient, clenching fists), then 84% of nursing home residents and 56% of intermediate care residents were rated as engaging in aggressive behaviors.

Burgio et al. (1988) had geriatric assistants fill out a Behavior Problem Survey for residents in their nursing home. The assistants rated 26% of the residents as showing tantrum-like behavior, 23% of the residents as showing noncompliance, 22% as engaging in verbal abuse, and 20% as engaging in physical aggression. Residents could be rated on more than one category, so the same residents undoubtedly had several of these behaviors.

These statistics tell the story that problem behaviors are a very frequent occurrence in long-term-care settings. Most of the residents in these settings apparently engage in some form of disruptive behavior at some time. The studies also found that the residents most likely to engage in problem behaviors were those with dementia (Bernier & Small, 1988; Zimmer et al., 1984). Of course, the way problem behaviors are defined will influence the rate of problems. Some of the studies with a high rate of problem behaviors had a very inclusive definition of what constituted problem behavior. Commonly defined problem behaviors may include: wandering, repetitive actions, language difficulties, altered sleep patterns, refusal to bathe, incontinence, anger or agitation, difficulty dressing, and eating difficulties (Schweiger & Huey, 1999). Problem behaviors can occur for many reasons—some easy to see and understand and some more subtle. We will be describing typical problem behaviors and the situations or conditions that can cause them. We will also discuss ways to deal with or solve such problems.

DIFFICULT BEHAVIOR PROBLEMS

The regular workload of caring for a demented or disabled person is a considerable job. The work is not only physically difficult but also mentally taxing. Even in the best of circumstances, there is also an emotional burden in caring for demented residents. Behavior problems just add to this load.

Many of these difficult behavior problems occur during times when direct, hands-on care is being given. One study (Jones, 1985) found that the highest occurrence of violent incidents was between 8:30 and 10:30 A.M. This is the time morning care is given in most long-term-care settings, the time when the most intense and prolonged interaction between resident and staff is likely to occur.

Residents often exhibit many behavior problems simultaneously. An agitated, verbally abusive resident may become physically abusive under certain circumstances. Residents who endanger themselves by refusing needed treatment may strike out and endanger others if they feel trapped and coerced by staff into accepting the treatment.

What are the difficult behavior problems faced each day by caregivers at home or in long-term-care settings? One common way of defining difficult behaviors is by including actions that are a danger to the residents themselves, behaviors that are a danger to those around them, and behaviors that are disturbing to others and disruptive of the routine (Ryden, 1989; Winger et al., 1987; Zimmer et al., 1984). Behavior problems can be classified into four main subtypes: physically aggressive behaviors, physically nonaggressive behaviors, verbally aggressive behaviors, verbally nonaggressive behavior (Cohen-Mansfield, Marx, & Rosenthal, 1989; Cohen-Mansfield, Werner, Watson, & Pasis, 1995 as cited in Cohen-Mansfield, 1999).

Agitation

A person who is agitated appears restless, anxious, and unhappy; this resident may be experiencing fatigue, pain, or discomfort (as from constipation), medication adverse effects, sensory overload, or feel lost or insecure from being in contact with unfamiliar places and people (Schweiger & Huey, 1999). Although agitation is broadly characterized—by anxiety and accompanied by restlessness—it occurs at some point in up to 80% of patients with dementia (Lehninger, Ravindran, & Stewart, 1998), and it may be expressed by restless, repetitive behaviors that the person appears to have little ability to control. These behaviors may take the form of verbalizations—either repetitive questions, calling out for help, shouting, or crying. They may take the form of repetitive physical behavior, such as swinging a crossed leg, pacing, picking or scratching the skin, or pounding on the tray of the gerichair. Agitation may appear as confusion between day and night, in which case a person may be relatively calm during the day but wakeful and upset during the night—hollering, wandering around the room, and resisting staff efforts to encourage quietness and sleep.

A resident who expresses agitation by being noisy can cause considerable disruption in a long-term-care setting. The behavior may be continuously calling for help, calling for some person from long ago, screaming, moaning, or sobbing. Such behavior is very wearing on both caregivers and other residents. It is also often very difficult to treat.

Aggression

Aggression can involve both verbal and physical abusiveness. Verbal abusiveness is very common and includes swearing, name-calling, unwarranted criticisms and accusations, and threats. Although we have all heard the old saying, "Sticks and stones will break my bones, but words will never hurt me," dealing with constant verbal abuse is very stressful for a caregiver. Physical abusiveness involves striking out, hitting, biting, kicking, pushing, and other actions that can injure others. Aggressiveness can also be directed at the self. Serious intentional self-injury and even suicide can occur in long-term-care settings.

Aggressive behavior that occurs during direct care activities is usually felt to be a reaction to the hands-on care. Furthermore, physical aggression is more common among moderately to severely demented individuals and occurs most often during daily care routines (Hoeffer et al., 1997 as cited in Allen-Burge et al., 1999). Aggression against other residents often occurs during a disagreement or argument. However, aggression does occur that appears relatively unprovoked. A resident may unexpectedly cover a roommate's head with a pillow or stick a cane out just in time to trip an innocent passerby. Some of this unprovoked aggression may result from the demented person's misidentification of the person or situation. If a caregiver becomes familiar with the resident's background and listens to what the resident has been saying, the caregiver may at times be able to predict when aggressive incidents will occur and intervene so as to prevent them.

Wandering

Wandering is a high-frequency behavior among demented individuals. Possible causes for wandering can include (but are not limited to): stress or physical discomfort, frustration, lack of stimulation, or searching for home or people from the past (Schweiger & Huey, 1999). Wandering puts the individual at great risk when, for instance, they leave the protected setting where they are living. Out in unknown territory, their impaired judgment and poor memory make them unable to cope. Wandering also leads to aggressive behavior between residents. When a wanderer enters another resident's room and touches another resident's possessions, aggressive incidents are apt to occur if the resident tries to protect the property. Wandering is significant enough and frequent enough that it has been given a separate chapter in this book (see chapter 8). There, a description of the behavior and management suggestions are presented in detail.

Other Aberrant Behaviors

Agitation, aggressiveness, and wandering are frequent aberrant behaviors in long-term-care settings. However, there are other less frequent behaviors that also cause problems to caregivers. Certain sexual behaviors, such as exposure or public masturbation, which are inappropriate but not necessarily aggressive, are examples (Ryden, 1989). In this category also are placed such offensive personal habits as nose blowing on sleeves or the hem of a dress, spitting on hands and then rubbing them. These are troublesome behaviors, which are disruptive and upsetting and need to be addressed in some way to restore harmony.

Suspiciousness/Paranoia

A fairly frequent situation that leads to problem behaviors in a demented resident is the resident's suspiciousness or misinterpretation of events. This can cause the resident to act in an agitated or aggressive manner. Caregivers in long-term-care facilities are constantly dealing with residents' complaints that their possessions have been stolen. Often the accusations are quite specific as to the suspected culprit, and the resident's accusations are very unpleasant. Usually the missing item is found in the "safe" place where the resident had put it in the first place, before the resident forgot where it was.

Persons with dementia also misidentify people in their environment and misinterpret what is happening. They often feel threatened by these misinterpretations and have the need to protect themselves. At times these misperceptions and faulty beliefs take on the strength of delusions. There are several typical scenarios that may be acted out, which often occur at certain points in the progressive decline of mental functioning in dementia (Cummings et al., 1987; Mace & Rabins, 1981).

For example, a man saw his image in a mirror in his home and did not recognize himself or even realize he was looking in a mirror. He started carrying a hammer around to protect himself from the "intruder," whom he suspected of carrying on an affair with his wife.

Other common delusions include false beliefs such as the following: the 86-year-old woman who physically attacked her 92-year-old husband for carrying on with the "young girls" in the (empty) apartment upstairs. The man who locked his wife of 40 years out of their apartment because he thought she was an imposter who looked just like his wife but was really a double. The woman who did not recognize her husband when she woke up one night and found him in bed with her. She panicked and called the police to save her from the stranger in her bed.

Older people, especially those living alone who are somewhat hard of hearing or mildly demented, often get the idea that there are others in the house with them. Sometimes these others are living in the cellar, sometimes in the attic. They come into the living space while the victim is asleep and disrupt things, take things, spread poisonous fumes, and so on. An older person with such beliefs often has all sorts of evidence to prove the point. Often some event has happened, such as a neighborhood teenage prank directed at the elderly person, which starts or exacerbates the situation. Such beliefs lead to extreme fear and discomfort on the part of the elderly person. Sufferers often seek help from the police, social service agencies, and anybody else they can call on at all hours of the day and night. Such beliefs usually disappear once these people are around others all the time, such as in a long-term-care setting. However, at times nursing home residents will also express delusional beliefs—someone is putting a powder in the bed to make them itch or is poisoning their food. It is important to remember that these expressions of paranoia are an attempt to respond to the stresses in life or to make sense of unusual events (e.g., things out of place, people not recognized). These paranoid ideas are beliefs the person has developed without proof—even if a caregiver provides evidence to disprove the idea, the caregiver is very unlikely to shake the person's belief (Winogrond, 1984). Therefore, it is not helpful to argue or point out inconsistencies. In addition, we may contribute to a resident's paranoia by our behaviors—for example, putting their medications into food to make them easier to swallow.

Resistiveness to Care

Many of the difficult behavior problems, such as agitation and aggressiveness, occur when direct care is being given. This is considered resistiveness to care. In addition to noisiness, verbal abusiveness, or striking out during care, a resident may rigidly stiffen the body, refusing to bend the joints to allow care to be given. This makes care much more difficult. Other residents may refuse food, liquids, and medications to the point of endangering their health. Still other residents may resist treatments and diagnostic tests. These are usually seen as behaviors endangering the well-being of the resident, but if in resisting care the resident also becomes aggressive to the caregiver, others are endangered as well.

CONDITIONS THAT LEAD TO PROBLEM BEHAVIORS

In dealing with any kind of problem, it helps to understand the background from which the problem arises. Often more than one factor is operating in the problem behavior of a particular resident. Once the possible causes are sorted out, caregivers can deal more directly with them and perhaps even prevent the behavior from occurring at all. The following are several reasons that explain why problem behaviors might be happening.

A Lifelong Personality Pattern

One reason for behavior that becomes a problem in an institutional setting is that a particular resident has always been a difficult person with whom to get along (Aronson, 1983; Morrant & Ablog, 1983). Many irascible, temperamental, or mean-spirited people are tolerated for years by their families or live by themselves. Their behavior is "dreadful," and they often have alienated and lost track of any family or friends they had. Once they become frail and elderly and are forced to come to a nursing home, they have a difficult adjustment to make. Their lifelong personality pattern interferes with adjusting to living with others and accepting care.

Mr. George, age 68, lived on the edge of town in a shack made of odds and ends of wood and covered with tarpaper. He made a living by picking up scrap metal and other junk and selling it. During some very cold weather, Mr. George was found in his shack, delirious with frostbitten, gangrenous toes. He recovered after partial amputation of his feet, but it was felt he could no longer live alone. He was placed in a nursing care facility. Once he had settled in, his habits and behaviors began to make the staff and other residents uncomfortable. His table manners were offensive, and his personal habits were careless. He had to be reminded frequently to change soiled clothes, button his shirt, zip his fly, and so on. He began collecting things in his room—old magazines and newspapers, broken jewelry and cans, and other things that had been discarded. Sometimes he was found with items the previous owner had not intended to throw away. He had great plans for why he needed these things and what he was going to do with them. He annoyed his roommates so much that he was eventually given a private room, which allowed him more space to accumulate stuff. Staff worried that Mr. George was creating a fire hazard, but other than insisting that he meet fire safety standards in storing his possessions, they were not sure what to do. He was ostracized by the other residents, disliked by many of the staff, and he just wanted to leave and go back to his home. However, that was considered too risky given his health, substandard home, and lack of any community supports. But it is doubtful that Mr. George could ever change his lifelong behavior pattern to comfortably live with others in an institution. His eccentricities must just be tolerated.

Likewise, people who have always prided themselves on their independence and self-reliance may find it particularly difficult to accept help with self-care tasks and may lash out at the caregiver.

Mrs. Dowd has arthritis and finds dressing very difficult. Especially in the morning, her shoulders are so stiff she can't get her nightshirt off or put on her blouse or dress. When the aide comes to help her, Mrs. Dowd swears at her and angrily criticizes everything the aide does. The aide found some garments that were designed for people with limited range of motion and which Mrs. Dowd can manage herself. Now her mornings are much more pleasant.

An approach that respects a resident's need for independence and that lessens the need for care may be helpful in these situations.

Reactions to Life Stress

Another reason for problem behavior in residents is their various reactions to life stresses. Residents may be experiencing grief, depression, frustration, loneliness, and isolation. These feelings can lead to problem behaviors. A person who is grieving (e.g., over the death of a spouse, the loss of a home, the loss of a former competent self) may have strong feelings of anger that lead the person to react with hostility or irritability to any caregiving approach. Often, problem behaviors may signify unmet needs and the resulting psychological or physiological distress in elderly individuals (Cohen-Mansfield, 1999). People who are depressed may whine and complain, become withdrawn, and make no attempt to help themselves.

Mrs. Henry's husband had died suddenly, and she sold her home and moved into a long-term-care facility. She also had serious health problems, including cancer, which appeared to be in remission. She was openly angry and hostile to most caregiving staff, frequently telling them how much she disliked them and demanding to be left alone. However, she was not completing self-care tasks, had several falls, and was not allowed to walk without supervision. She would not do anything for herself, including eating, drinking, or going to the bathroom. Mrs. Henry became severely constipated but still refused to cooperate with any treatment. Her level of anger and unhappiness was so great that she perversely and with great willpower made life as miserable as possible for herself and those around her.

People reacting to losses in this way seemingly work hard to make everyone around them feel as miserable as they do.

People sometimes respond to frustration by "acting out." All people act out at times. Acting out means directing outward what we feel inside. When something (for instance, the vacuum cleaner) doesn't work the way we want it to, we may throw it down or give it a kick out of sheer frustration. Residents who act out during personal care may be responding to the frustration of no longer being able to do these things for themselves.

Feelings of loneliness and isolation can lead to desperation and despair. This may be seen in constant attention seeking from staff.

Mrs. Walters was always at the nurses' station, constantly asking, "What should I do now?"

Feelings of loneliness and isolation can also lead to withdrawal, which, though less noticeable than constant attention-seeking behavior, may be a greater problem in the long run. People who withdraw may isolate themselves even more and begin to lose the will to take care of themselves, giving up to illness and physical decline.

Another reaction to life stress is to become suspicious and paranoid about what is happening around you. Sometimes because of cognitive impairment or poor hearing, you don't understand what is happening around you, and the only reasonable explanation is the unacceptable one of failing mentally. It is easier to explain what is happening by blaming others for plotting to make things difficult than to accept changes in yourself. When memory is regressing toward childhood, as it often seems to do in Alzheimer's disease, you may believe you are 40 years old instead of 80. The elderly woman who claims to be your wife must be an imposter who has kidnapped your real wife, who you remember as she was at age 35. When a resident is experiencing chronic, progressive, degenerative diseases, it is reasonable to blame the losses on what was eaten or drunk. From that belief, it is a short step to feeling that somebody is putting poison in the food or water. How else can these individuals explain why they are feeling worse and worse? Residents who develop such suspicions often try to gain some control over their situation by acting on these beliefs. They may refuse all food unless it is in a closed package, such as a closed carton of milk or intact package of cookies. This can severely tax a caregiver's ingenuity for providing a balanced diet.

Dementing Illness

As might be expected, another source of behavior problems in long-term-care residents is dementing illness. Persons with dementia exhibit many problem behaviors—disorientation, wandering (because they may feel lost or in the wrong place), not knowing their way around (so they don't remember where the bathroom is), poor impulse control (being affectionate with the wrong people), combativeness, and acting in other ways that are not socially acceptable.

One characteristic of persons with brain damage is a tendency towards exhibiting a "catastrophic reaction" (Mace & Rabins, 1981). When people respond to a seemingly minor event as if it were a catastrophe (with rage, tears, verbal and physical acting out, running away), they are exhibiting a catastrophic reaction. Often a caregiver is taken by surprise when such a reaction occurs.

Miss Trimble was confused and forgetful but wanted to stay in her own apartment. A social service agency had provided her with daily personal care aides to help her manage the tasks of daily living. Miss Trimble didn't always remember who the aides were or what they were doing in her apartment, but the aides were usually able to satisfy her with an explanation, and she accepted their help. For a change of scene, one day an aide decided to take Miss Trimble shopping. They went to a newly opened supermarket that had all the latest features. Once in the store, Miss Trimble became more and more confused. As the aide took her arm to guide her to another display, Miss Trimble yelled, "Who are you? Let go of me at once!" and swung her purse at the aide, knocking off the aide's glasses. It took some time to calm Miss Trimble down and get her back to the safe territory of her familiar apartment. In analyzing this event afterward, it is apparent that Miss Trimble was being asked to do something more complicated than she could handle. She was overwhelmed by too many demands or too many stimuli in an unfamiliar environment.

The best way to deal with catastrophic reactions is to figure out the circumstances that cause them in a resident and then avoid those circumstances. For instance, some activities that are too difficult for the resident to accomplish may cause the resident to storm and cry. Simplify a task by breaking it down into small steps so the resident won't be overwhelmed by the entire sequence all at once. One example is the task of dressing. Instead of telling a resident to "get dressed," a phrase that may no longer have meaning, caregivers must make their statements much more specific. First the caregiver could say, "Put on your shirt." The caregiver may even have to be more specific than this by saying, "Pick up your shirt. Put your arm in the armhole." You can also simplify the environment so that the resident is not confronted by too many activities going on at once. The caregiver should turn off the television set when feeding a person, for instance. Also, it is important to be very calm when a catastrophic reaction occurs and distract the individual, taking the person slowly away from the frustrating situation.

Sundown Syndrome

A problem that is often seen in dementia residents but also may occur in nondemented residents is sundown syndrome. This syndrome refers to the change in resident behavior that is often observed close to the time the sun goes down. Many staff in long-term-care facilities have noticed that residents' behavior seems to get worse at the end of the day. There are many reasons suggested for why this might be so. Decreased levels of light could be disorienting, as residents can't see familiar things as well. A resident may be overtired and thus behaves worse. The resident may be experiencing mild delirium because of dehydration, drug effects, or circulatory problems worsened by fatigue. The bustle of shift change is also overstimulating. Probably a combination of these factors leads to the sundown syndrome.

Nighttime or Sleep Problems

Perhaps related to sundown syndrome are nighttime problems affecting many dementia residents; in fact, up to 70% of individuals with dementia exhibit sleep problems (Lehninger et al., 1998). At times residents who are quiet and easily managed during the day become noisy, combative, and noncompliant at night. The problem might be a disruption of the daily cycle where the person is disoriented to time of day and is up and dressed at 2:00 A.M., insisting it is time for breakfast. At other times the person may be responding to an event the person has dreamed about and doesn't realize it has been a dream. The borderline between sleep and waking is a very vulnerable time for the brain. Most of us have had experiences of waking up suddenly by a telephone ringing and being confused for a short time, perhaps not even responding normally. For a demented person, this rather common experience may be exaggerated and prolonged by the already impaired functioning of the brain. The lower levels of sensory stimulation at night (less light, quieter) may add to the disorientation.

Physical Environment

There are reasons for residents' problem behaviors that involve unclear aspects of the physical environment. The physical setting may provide circumstances, which, coupled with residents' sensory impairments and dementia, may lead to disordered behavior. One example of this is shiny floors. Some residents can perceive this shininess as puddles. Sometimes they urinate in these "puddles," reasoning that since they don't know where the bathroom is and since there is already water there, they may as well add to it. Likewise, the public address system can lead to delusional behavior on the part of some residents, who believe that they are being called or that someone is talking to them. Environmental change is another circumstance that can lead to increased problem behavior. Changes in residents' rooms or roommates, or sending residents to the emergency room or hospital, can impose a great deal of stress and lead to problem behavior.

Caregiver Stress

A final possible cause of problem behavior in residents is the moods and actions of people in their environment including caregivers, coupled with residents' sensitivity to emotional undertones and tensions. There have been multiple studies about behavior problems in residents in long-term care that result in stress among the staff caring for them (Astrom, Nilsson, Norberg, & Winblad, 1990; Clinton, Moyle, Weir, & Edwards, 1995; Everitt, Fields, Soumerai, & Avorn, 1991 as cited in Cohen-Mansfield, 1999). There are numerous reasons for tensions and negative feelings in the work setting. Some are caused by the institution itself. For example, the inspectors are coming, layoffs are threatened, and a well-liked supervisor is being replaced by one who has the reputation of being an ogre. Residents seem to pick up on these tensions and respond as if they also are under stress with problem behaviors. This particular source of behavior problems can best be dealt with by a certain degree of openness and information about the underlying institutional problems and reassurance of continued care and concern for the well-being of the residents.

There is a wide range of variability among response and adaptation to stressors among caregivers; in caregiving research, studies find that people in similar situations react in highly different ways (Zarit, 1994 as cited in Zarit, 1996). Differences in caregivers' response may be caused by the type of illness, the level of care required, the available support system, and the relationship of the caregiver tot he patient (Watson, Modeste, Catolico, & Crouch, 1998). Other reasons for staff tensions are personal—poor sleep, a hangover, a family crisis. Some reasons for tension have to do with a caregiver's fear of or dislike of a resident. As discussed elsewhere in this book, residents are sensitive to another person's moods and manner of approach. The caregiver's awareness of his or her own tension, fear, or irritability is vital. These feelings need to be dealt with before going in to care for a resident—by confiding in a friend, getting support from a supervisor, laughing more at one's self, taking a few deep breaths, and putting the problem in perspective.

Another factor in caregiver stress is that the job itself is stressful. Because of experiences on the job, caregivers see the sickest, weakest, frailest, and most seriously impaired older adults. Caring for them is very hard work, both physically and emotionally. It is also easy to be fearful in this situation, worrying about one's own safety and one's own old age. At times, fear may cause caregivers to avoid their residents, to spend less time with them, talk to them less, touch them less. We all tend to avoid what causes us stress. It's only natural. But we hope with increased awareness and understanding as a result of reading this book, caregivers will overcome such fears and not allow them to affect job performance and satisfaction.

SOLVING DIFFICULT PROBLEMS

Developing Empathy

One approach to managing difficult behavior problems is to study the resident and the circumstances that lead to the problems and see what can be changed to avoid the behavior in the future. This involves developing empathy or understanding of the resident. The caregiver must make an effort to mentally "walk in the resident's shoes" for a time to try to understand things from the resident's perspective. It also involves becoming more aware of personal behaviors and attitudes on the part of the caregiver—noticing not only what the caregiver might be doing that makes the situation worse, but also what the caregiver does that makes the situation better. If one staff member is always successful in managing a resident, find out what the person does and try to copy it. Also, it is important to keep an objective viewpoint about what the resident says or does. Caregivers cannot allow themselves to take personally the insults or actions of a difficult resident. If caregivers do take these things personally, it not only interferes with their ability to work with the resident, but it adds to their stress level and is not healthy for them. With effort, if it doesn't come naturally, caregivers can make a conscious decision not to take to heart the insults and curses an agitated resident might direct toward them. They are not really meant for the caregivers personally. Many times residents reserve the most hateful insults and criticisms for the caregivers they admire the most. The negative behavior is a reflection of their own unhappiness and self-hate.

An important circumstance to be aware of occurs when demented residents are confused and misidentify individuals and misinterpret their environment.

Mr. Woodly, 67 and newly admitted to the facility, hit a staff member over the head with a vase as the staff member was helping an elderly woman resident to bed. Mr. Woodly had earlier in the day referred to the woman as his mother, had been nice to her, and had objected to staff giving her care. Before entering the long-term-care facility, Mr. Woodly had once physically threatened his wife, insisting she was a stranger and must leave the house. Although it probably would not have helped the situation to persuade Mr. Woodly of his error in thinking of the woman resident as his mother, the caregiver's awareness of his mistaken belief and of his threats of violence might have made the caregiver take more precautions around him. The caregiver could have distracted him in another part of the unit while care was being given to the female resident, until he became more accepting of the situation.

Inappropriate sexual behaviors on the part of the residents are another area where it is important for the caregivers to know themselves and how they come across to residents.

The mental health consultant was called in to see Mr. Able, an 86-year-old resident of a nursing home, because he was making sexual advances to female aides and nurses. Mr. Able was interviewed with the nurse on the unit, who said to him, "Now you know, honey, we can't have this kind of behavior." It was pointed out that there was a mixed message in that statement. If the resident was frequently called "honey" and "dear" by the nurses—terms usually reserved for sweethearts and intimate partners—he might have some right to be confused.

Although, as authors, we emphasize over and over the importance of being warm and friendly to residents, the importance of touching them and helping them feel they are well-liked and worthwhile human beings, it is also important to recognize the need to avoid the suggestion of sexual provocativeness in this approach.

Psychoactive Medications

One approach for handling problem behaviors is with psychoactive medication (Lehninger et al., 1998; Raskind, Risse, & Lampe, 1987; Reisberg et al., 1987; Thomas, 1988).

There are several classes of psychoactive drugs used to control behavior. The physician will choose to prescribe a certain class of drug and a specific drug based on the particular type of behavior problem the resident is displaying. The caregiver's careful observation and reporting of resident behavior is important here. One class of drugs is the major tranquilizers, also known as antipsychotic drugs or neuroleptics. This class of drugs includes Thorazine, Mellaril, Haldol, Prolixin, Navane, and several others. Newer antipsychotic medications, called atypical antipsychotics, include Clozaril, Resperidol, and Xyprexia. The minor tranquilizers comprise another class of drugs. These are also known as antianxiety agents. Many of the drugs in this classification are known chemically as benzodiazepines and include Valium, Xanax, Serax, and Ativan. Buspar is an antianxiety drug that is not a benzodiazepine. Antidepressants constitute another class of psychoactive medications. These include selective serotonin reuptake inhibitors (SSRIs) and tricyclic antidepressants. Another type of antidepressant, the monoamine oxidase inhibitors (MAOI), such as Nardil and Parnate, are also available for use. Lithium is a drug used in the treatment of manic-depression. Another class of psychoactive medication often prescribed in nursing homes is sedative-hypnotics. Restoril, Dalmane, Ambien, and Halcion are all popularly prescribed to induce sleep. Chloral hydrate is noted by many physicians to be a safe, effective drug to bring on sleep in the elderly (Jenike, 1989).

Anticholinergic drugs (Artane, Cogentin) are a class of drugs often given to counteract some of the side effects of the major tranquilizers.

A drug such as Benadryl is sometimes prescribed because of its sedative, calming effect. There has been some research showing that the use of beta-blockers such as Inderal can be effective in controlling agitation problems (Jenike, 1989; Salzman, 1987). Antiseizure medications such as Tegretol and Depakote are sometimes used to help stabilize mood in persons with or without a seizure disorder.

Studies that have been done to evaluate the effects of psychoactive drugs on the demented elderly have generally shown real but limited value from their use (Barnes et al., 1982; Jenike, 1989; Raskind et al., 1987). The major tranquilizers have been found to be quite effective for such problems as hallucinations, paranoid delusions, agitation, and aggressiveness (Raskind et al., 1987; Salzman, 1987; Thomas, 1988). Expert consensus guidelines (Anonymous, 1998) advocate Risperdol as the agent of first choice. Antidepressants can offer very effective treatment for depression. The minor tranquilizers are often given for anxiety and agitation. They frequently do have a calming effect for mild anxiety and agitation, but are not as effective as major tranquilizers for more severe symptoms (Salzman, 1987); in fact, diazepam (Valium) was frequently given in large doses until behavior was controlled; however, this approach is no longer used because of the drug's deleterious side effects (e.g., oversedation, impaired cognitive function, and rebound agitation) (Tappen, 1997). The sedative-hypnotics will usually bring on sleep and can be used effectively over the short term to help reestablish a suitable sleep pattern. However, they should not be prescribed on a long-term basis as they are quite addictive.

However, all of these medications have side effects and unwanted actions that make their use somewhat of a problem with the elderly. In the first place, elders usually tolerate very small doses of these drugs, much smaller doses than physicians would prescribe for younger patients; second, older people require lower doses of medication as they have an increased sensitivity to drugs, changes in distribution of fat throughout the body, and slower clearance and elimination of many drugs (Tappen, 1997). This is especially true for people with dementia, who often seem particularly vulnerable to the adverse effects of these drugs even in very small amounts.

SIDE EFFECTS OF PSYCHOACTIVE MEDICATIONS

What are some of the most significant side effects of psychoactive medications? One of the most frequent side effects is excessive sedation

(Salzman, 1987). Because one of the major ways the drugs work is through sedation, it is necessary to find just the right dose to induce the desired calming effect without causing excessive sleepiness and stupor (Thomas, 1988). If residents are too sedated, they may become more confused, which can lead to increased agitation, thus contradicting the desired effect of the drug. Also, an overly sedated resident may not eat as well or move around as much, leading to a greater risk of overall physical decline.

Other side effects include orthostatic hypotension—a sudden drop in blood pressure when transferring from a sitting to a standing position. This can lead to an increased risk of falls and subsequent fractures. A resident may develop drug-induced symptoms of Parkinson's disease with tremors and rigidity that can be very upsetting. Residents also may develop anticholinergic side effects, which include dry mouth, blurred vision, urinary retention, constipation, confusion, poor memory, and difficulty learning new things. Because the latter are also major symptoms of dementia, taking a drug that makes these symptoms worse is counterproductive.

A major risk of taking neuroleptic medications is tardive dyskinesia. This is a movement disorder that develops as a result of taking these drugs. The disorder involves abnormal movements or tremors of the mouth or limbs and can be very unpleasant to the sufferer, interfering with walking, eating, and sitting still. Personal appearance is also very unpleasant, as the afflicted person is constantly jutting out the tongue, contorting the face, and flailing arms. Drs. Lehninger, Ravindran, and Stewert (1998) assert that several studies suggest that wandering might be aggravated by neuroleptic-induced motor restlessness (akathisia).

Benzodiazepines may produce paradoxical agitation (an effect opposite to what the drug intended), incontinence, confusion, and instability in older residents (Winograd & Jarvik, 1986). Persons with dementia may be particularly susceptible to loss of control over aggressive impulses when taking benzodiazepines (Jenike, 1989). These drugs also can be addictive and should not be discontinued suddenly in a person who has been using them for a long time.

Because many of the drugs described previously have similar calming effects on behavior, physicians usually prescribe a given drug on the basis of which side effects the particular resident can best tolerate. However, it is difficult to predict exactly which side effects or adverse reactions a person might experience. Therefore, a resident taking a new medication needs to be carefully observed. The new drug should be suspected should any unusual behavior or symptoms occur. The new drug may also be interacting with other medications the resident is taking, causing a polypharmacy effect, which can have many harmful consequences. Because there are many drugs with similar desirable effects, if a resident experiences a bad reaction to one medication, another can be tried. Often the physician will need to try several different psychoactive drugs before finding one that produces a beneficial effect with a minimum of side effects (Jenike, 1989).

After consideration, it would seem that psychoactive medications should be used sparingly with elderly residents. Because of their excessive sedation in some cases and utility in controlling agitation and aggression, they are sometimes called "chemical restraints." Although they can in fact help control some problem behaviors, it is recommended that the medications be prescribed carefully and that their use be time limited (Sherman, 1988; Thomas, 1988). Using psychoactive medications is just one approach to managing problem behaviors of agitation, aggressiveness, paranoia, resistiveness to care, and other aberrant actions. Other nondrug measures must also be used to successfully help residents. These include problem solving, self-awareness, modifying and simplifying the physical environment, and using calming communication techniques to gain the resident's trust and prevent catastrophic reactions and other problem behaviors from occurring.

DEVELOPING A TREATMENT PLAN

Problem behaviors should be assessed and treated whether the resident is in a hospital, long-term-care facility, or home; one approach to dealing with problem behavior is to develop a plan with other members of the health care team to address the problem. Such a plan is often called a "treatment plan" or an "resident care plan." This plan is intended to guide the care that the individual resident receives (Ouslander, Osterweil, & Morley, 1997). The first step in developing such a strategy is to identify the problem (Zarit, Orr, & Zarit, 1985). Cohen and Pushkar (1999) note that individuals with dementia will often spend time in acute hospital settings and their special needs must be addressed if they are to be discharged back home; therefore, correct identification of the problem is essential in a resident's care.

For instance, is the problem that Mr. Finney insists on urinating in the corner of the hallway? Or is the problem that Mr. Finney is disoriented, has no idea where the bathroom is located, and is doing his best to be discreet?

When you have decided how to define the problem, you must find out when and how often it occurs. Keeping a log or a daily record for a short while can help you find out the frequency of problem behaviors and the usual circumstances that accompany these behaviors (Zarit et al., 1985). Knowing how often the problem behavior actually occurs and the circumstances that accompany it can help the caregiver plan strategies for managing the behavior. The caregiver can discover the antecedents, or what circumstances come before the behavior—and what consequences follow the behavior. This will help determine the underlying causes of the problem.

The next step is deciding on a goal or objective. How should the resident act? What behavior is desirable in place of the problem behavior? Once a goal is identified, the next step is to decide how to change things—what strategies or methods will establish the new, desirable behavior? The caregiver should think of several different approaches or strategies, consider the advantages and disadvantages of each approach, and then choose the one with the most advantages and least disadvantages to try initially.

It is important that a treatment plan be written down. Everyone who works with the resident can read it and know the objectives and interventions for this particular resident. Also, a written plan allows for review of the treatment to determine what is working and to decide if the goal has been met. The goal should be stated in such a way as to determine when it has been accomplished. In other words, it should be written in measurable terms. Also, the methods should be specific as to what is going to be done, who is going to be responsible for doing it, and when it is going to be done (e.g., time of day, frequency, and date to be accomplished).

Problem solving is often a matter of trial and error. Frequently, the strategy or plan that has been implemented must be revised or discarded and another strategy tried. It is important to keep a problem-solving frame of mind. If something does not work at first, the caregiver should analyze the situation and try new strategies based on the analysis. The exercises in this chapter provide practice in the procedures of treatment planning and problem solving.

The Resident Assessment Instrument

An invaluable tool now common in long-term-care facilities—used to gather data for treatment and resident care plans—is the Resident Assessment Instrument (RAI) with its major components, the Minimum Data Set (MDS) and Resident Assessment Protocols (RAP). The Nursing Home Reform Act in the Omnibus Budget Reconciliation Act of 1987 (OBRA-87) is responsible for long-term-care facilities' usage of the RAI, which is enforced by the Health Care Financing Administration (HCFA) (Cox, 1998); the RAI with its MDS has been used by all Medicare- and Medicaid-certified nursing homes since 1991, as a result of the mandate stipulated by Medicare and Medicaid reimbursement (Bernabei et al., 1999). Bernabei et al., (1999) assert that the introduction of the MDS has been responsible for improving the accuracy and comprehensiveness of nursing home data and provides a sensitive measure of residents' functional change over time.

The purpose of the RAI is to improve individual care planning and the quality of care delivered in nursing homes (Hansebo, Kihlgren, Ljunggren, & Winblad, 1998). The MDS—a 284-item instrument used to assess the medical, psychological, and social characteristics of nursing home residents—is a systematic attempt to monitor the status and progress of residents (Lawton et al., 1998). This instrument is implemented at the time of admission—the MDS must be completed within 14 days of admission (Ouslander et al., 1997)—and annually, with periodic full and/or partial updates as determined by time and possible changed condition of the resident (Lawton et al., 1998). The Instrument takes approximately 60 to 90 minutes to complete, facilitates communication across disciplines, and uses numerous sources of information (e.g., patient, relatives, staff and medical/nursing records) (Hansebo et al., 1998). Furthermore, completion of the MDS identifies "triggers" that prompt further assessment of specific areas that indicate poor functioning by use of a RAP (Cox, 1998) in care planning (e.g., delirium, dementia, problem behaviors, restraints, dementia, incontinence). The RAP is an essential component of the identified poor functioning areas because it provides recommendations for further assessment, care planning, and examines the cause(s) of existing problems and prompts a plan of action. From these elements, care planning—problem identification, goals and plans of actions (approaches)—may be implemented.

HELPFUL HINTS FOR MANAGING DIFFICULT BEHAVIOR PROBLEMS

The following are suggestions, approaches, and strategies for handling difficult behavior problems in demented persons. These ideas have been gathered from various sources, including books on caring for dementia residents (Gwyther, 1985; Mace & Rabins, 1981; Tappen, 1997), published literature (Lehninger et al., 1999; Schweiger & Huey, 1999) and from experienced caregivers of dementia residents. First, there are general suggestions that can be applied to many problem behaviors, including agitation, anger and aggressiveness, wandering, suspiciousness, and other aberrant behaviors. Following the general suggestions are more specific suggestions pertinent to specific problem behaviors.

General Suggestions for Solving Problem Behaviors

1. Have the resident medically evaluated—look for a physical reason for a change or intensification of behavior.
2. Keep a diary or log for a few days—this could pinpoint the causes or consequences of the behavior, which could then be modified to change the behavior.
3. Check the physical discomfort of the resident—is the person hungry, fatigued, thirsty, in pain, too hot or too cold, constipated, experiencing sensory overload?
4. Simplify the environment—reduce frustration and overstimulation.
5. Anticipate problem situations—plan to avoid or minimize them. Plan rest periods to avoid fatigue. Maintain a consistent routine. Keep the environment quiet and uncluttered. Plan simple, success-oriented activities.
6. Recognize the need for a feeling of being in control—allow choices, and involve the resident in decision making.
7. Be creative—staff bothered by a male resident's "roaming hands" had him place his hands on the top of his head before providing personal care.

Suggestions for Handling Agitation

1. Evaluate the medication regimen—look for possible adverse side effects of medication.

2. Try music—rhythmic music, such as classical guitar or harpsi-chord, may be more calming than violin or orchestral music.
3. Find some constructive task for the person to do—folding towels, sorting cards, gardening.
4. Reduce stimulation in the environment.
5. Simplify tasks—break tasks down into their simplest steps.
6. Approach the resident in a calm, gentle manner—the caregiver's calmness will help the resident become calm. If the resident has made an error, provide reassurance and focus his/her attention elsewhere.

Suggestions for Handling Anger and Aggressiveness

1. Keep daily routine consistent—avoid surprises.
2. Protect residents from hurting themselves—remove sharp objects and other possible weapons from the environment.
3. Remove the resident from the stressful environment—gently lead the person away, talking in a calm, soothing voice tone.
4. Distract the individual—try a favorite activity or a food treat.
5. Avoid reasoning or asking questions the person may have trouble answering—try a gentle, calming touch.
6. Make sure the resident gets regular exercise—this could relieve tension.
7. Be aware of nonverbal communications—the caregiver should try to appear calm and confident, and avoid appearing angry or impatient. The caregiver should use feeling identification with the resident.
8. If the physically threatening behavior of the resident puts the caregiver in danger of being hurt, leave the scene; get help.

Suggestions for Handling Wandering

1. Allow the person to wander—make the environment safe and secure.
2. Have the person wear an identification bracelet. Keep a picture of the resident on file. Introduce the resident to neighbors and storeowners in the area.

3. Help these individuals find their way around the environment—clearly label rooms with printed signs or pictures. Place familiar objects and furniture in the surroundings.
4. Take the person for a walk, outside if possible.
5. Provide another activity—distract the person from wandering, limiting activities to 30 minutes. "Trigger" items should be removed from residents view (e.g., hat, coat, purse, car keys).
6. Reassure wandering residents about where they are, why they are there, and that their families know where to find them. Use a calm, friendly voice tone.
7. Use monitoring devices if possible to track patients.

Suggestions for Sundowning/Nighttime Restlessness

1. Be sure there is adequate lighting in the evening. Provide nightlights and a well-lit path to the bathroom. Take the resident to the bathroom before bed.
2. Restrict caffeine and alcohol intake. Also, avoid stimulant and diuretic medications in the evening.
3. Reduce environmental activity at end of day. Reduce the bustle of shift change. Avoid overstimulating programs.
4. Establish a set bedtime routine. Discourage excessive napping during the day, although to avoid fatigue, a short midday nap may be helpful.
5. Provide an opportunity for healthy exercise during the day. A walk, preferably outside, is a good idea.
6. Provide comforting things for the resident—a soft stuffed animal, enjoyable music, a comforting food treat.

Suggestions for Handling Suspiciousness

1. Do not whisper to someone else in front of the person. Do not discuss the resident as if the person were not present.
2. Help look for a missing item—know the resident's usual hiding places, and look there first.
3. Reduce potential hiding places by eliminating clutter and locking unused areas. Keep an extra set of frequently lost items. Check wastebaskets before emptying.

4. Avoid responding defensively to accusations. Avoid arguing or providing a lengthy explanation—be calm and reassuring. Recognize the underlying fear or feeling of loss of control.

Suggestions for Handling Resistiveness to Care

1. Use a calm, matter-of-fact approach—give simple instructions, step by step.
2. Consider privacy issues in bathing, toileting—provide for the privacy needs of residents.
3. Offer the residents some choice. Let the residents feel they have some control. Let them do what they can for themselves, even if it takes more time. Let them make their own decisions, if possible, about when an activity should be scheduled.
4. Give the person something constructive to do while care is being given—have the person hold a washcloth during bathing, for instance.
5. Make the caregiving time special and pleasant using soft music, scented lotions, or gentle massage. Try telling an amusing story, or get the resident to talk about a particular interest during care.
6. Be aware of nonverbal communications. The caregiver should avoid appearing angry, tense, or afraid of the resident. The caregiver should take time to relax and get in a good frame of mind before approaching the resident who is difficult to care for.

SUMMARY

This chapter has described some of the difficult problem behaviors often seen in residents with dementia in long-term-care settings: agitation, aggression, paranoia, resistiveness to care, and other common aberrant behaviors. The reasons underlying these problems have been examined, including a lifelong personality pattern, reactions to life stress, dementing illness, sundown syndrome, the physical environment, and caregiver stress. Suggested steps to take to solve these problems include better self-awareness on the part of the caregiver and better understanding of the residents, medications, and treatment planning approaches. A list of helpful hints in managing problem behaviors is also included.

LEARNING EXERCISES

Analyze and develop a treatment plan for the following cases:

1. "What time is it?" Mr. McDonald asks. You tell him, as you hurry from his room. Two minutes later, Mr. McDonald walks up to the nurses' station. "What time is it?" You tell him, feeling annoyed. In fact, Mr. McDonald annoys all the staff with his incessant questioning. Everyone avoids him whenever possible. Even other residents of the nursing home know to keep their distance. And the situation just seems to be getting worse.

   • What is the immediate problem?
   • What are the underlying reasons for the problem?
   • How do you think this makes the caregiver feel?
   • What will be the treatment plan?

2. Everyone is afraid of Mr. Howard. Although he is 87 and looks quite frail, he is surprisingly strong when he wants to be. He is unsteady on his feet and is only supposed to walk with staff supervision and assistance. But Mr. Howard usually climbs over the bed rails at night to roam the halls. He yells and swears at staff who bring his meals and medications. He resists personal care, and it is a constant battle to keep him clean and groomed.
   Mr. Howard particularly hates baths, insisting that he just had one even though the caregiver knows he did not. Last night, on the evening shift, he kicked an aide in the ribs when he was being changed for bed. The aide couldn't finish her shift and may have cracked ribs. Mr. Howard has swung at the caregiver when he was given care, but so far the caregiver has not been hit. He has succeeded in pinching the caregiver, however. Today, because of the incident last night, staff is refusing to approach Mr. Howard to give him the bath he badly needs. What should the caregiver do about Mr. Howard's bath today, and what should the caregiver do about managing his abusiveness?

   • What is the immediate problem?
   • What are the underlying reasons for the problem?
   • How do you think this makes the caregiver feel?
   • Treatment plan?

3. Sarah Wilson is a delightful resident, usually smiling and helpful. She always does errands for the other residents. However, she usually won't attend activities or parties. Although the staff knows Sarah has family living in the area, they rarely come to visit her. When the staff question Sarah about why she won't attend social events, she says, "I'm waiting for my daughter. I don't want to miss her when she comes." One day a troubling incident occurs. Mrs. Wilson put all her clothes in some paper bags and sat by the front door of the nursing home with them. She says to the caregiver, "I told my daughter I want to go home. She'll be here soon to pick me up." How would you deal with the situation, immediately and in the long run?

   • What is the immediate problem?
   • What are the underlying reasons for the problem?
   • How does it make you feel?
   • Treatment plan?

4. You are a staff member working the evening shift. Late in your shift, you hear a commotion in Mr. Brown's room. When you investigate, you find that Mrs. Allen has entered his room and crawled into bed with him. Everybody in the room is very upset— Mr. Brown is indignant, his roommate is annoyed at having been awakened; and Mrs. Allen is very confused and tearful. She keeps repeating, "Ralph," the name of her husband who died 3 years ago. This is not the first time that Mrs. Allen has gotten into someone else's bed. Her family, when informed in the past of this behavior, was very embarrassed, saying she had not acted that way before. Right now you have three very upset people on your hands. What do you do immediately and in the long run?

   • What is the immediate problem?
   • What are the underlying reasons for the problem?
   • How does it make you feel?
   • Treatment plan?

SUGGESTED ANSWERS

1. The following are suggested answers to the case of Mr. Mc-Donald.

- Immediate problem: Mr. McDonald bothers everyone with his continual questioning.
- Underlying reasons: Mr. McDonald wants attention, feels insecure. Because of his memory problem, he is not sure of himself. He may have an inability to stop the questions because of his dementia. He may also believe he has important appointments to keep, as he did in his former job. He has gotten into a vicious cycle of alienating people so that he can't get social stimulation, which might improve his condition.
- How it makes staff feel: They feel impatient, not wanting him near.
- Treatment plan:
  Goal: Increase the resident's appropriate interaction with others, and decrease his isolation.
  Method: The staff should reassure Mr. McDonald by saying, "We'll take care of you; we like you," with a friendly touch to emphasize this. They should try to find meaningful activities for him, such as group exercises, crafts, or making friends with another resident.

2. The following are suggested answers to the case of Mr. Howard.

- Immediate problem: Mr. Howard has body odor, is abusive, and can hurt you.
- Underlying reasons: He has moderate dementia, causing disinhibition. With brain damage, he may be unable to control his impulses. He resents being in this kind of place and is uncomfortable having people give such personal care.
- How it makes staff feel: They feel scared, disgusted, and incompetent to handle the situation.
- Treatment plan:
  Goal: Have patient accept baths without combativeness.
  Method: Staff should see if Mr. Howard could be bathed by a male aide. The aide should show Mr. Howard that he doesn't intimidate him. Staff should use a nonthreatening (open, relaxed) posture when approaching him and use a calm, self-confident, friendly voice, explaining what they are doing. Their attitude will influence how he treats them. They should give Mr. Howard some control over his situation. Let him pick the

time of day he wants to be bathed, for example. They should use behavior modification—praise him when he acts normally, try to ignore him when he doesn't. Staff should find out what he likes—maybe hard candies—and see if they can give him one when he acts nicely. They should distract Mr. Howard, give him a task to do during bath time (holding a wash cloth) while they proceed with their task.

3. The following are suggested answers to the case of Mrs. Wilson.

- Immediate problem: Mrs. Wilson is all packed up and ready to leave, and you must convince her to unpack without getting her too upset.
- Underlying reasons: She is lonely, has had no family visits recently, and hasn't made close friends in the facility.
- How it makes staff feel: They feel pity and concern, and worry that she'll create a scene.
- Treatment plan:
  Goal: Increase the resident's socialization within the home.
  Method: Staff should identify Mrs. Wilson's feelings—saying, for example, "I guess your home is very important to you, and your family is very important to you." To reassure her, a staff member should hold her hand (Indian handshake) or give her a hug. Staff should ask Mrs. Wilson to postpone leaving, as it is getting late. Ask the nurse supervisor to contact the social worker to get the family in. Mrs. Wilson should be told to write her family a letter, which the caregiver will mail for her, or Mrs. Wilson should be helped to phone her family. Staff should encourage her to attend activities in the facility. Staff should ask her to befriend or help with a frailer resident.

4. The following are suggested answers to the case of Mrs. Allen.

- Immediate problem: Three people are upset.
- Underlying reasons: Mrs. Allen gets into bed with someone she thinks is her husband, perhaps because of unresolved grief, loneliness, and dementia. Sundown syndrome might be affecting her.
- How it makes staff feel: Staff may interpret what has been going on as a sexual situation, and this makes them feel embarrassed.

However, Mrs. Allen is probably seeking reassurance and comfort rather then sexual activity.
- Treatment plan:
  Goal: Increase the resident's awareness of the location of her own bed, and help the resident accept the loss of her husband. *Method*: The caregiver should calm everybody down with a soothing voice tone. Mrs. Allen should be walked back to her room, perhaps with an arm around her shoulder. The incident should be reported to the charge nurse on the floor in an objective manner. The caregiver should pay more attention to Mrs. Allen and give her more touch and something to hug at night, such as a stuffed animal. Volunteer visits might be arranged if possible. For sundown syndrome, the caregiver should check if her behavior is worse at night. The caregiver should give her a little extra attention at night and talk with her about her husband. Her nightlight might be left on. The caregiver should respect confidentiality, and not joke with others about what happened.

POSTTEST

Place a "T" before true statements, an "F" before false statements, and a question mark before those you don't know.

_____ 1. Some residents who cause problems during personal care are too independent to accept help in such tasks.

_____ 2. The decreased light levels and confusion of staff changes toward the end of the day may contribute to problem behavior in some residents.

_____ 3. When residents lash out or cry over a seemingly insignificant event, they may be experiencing a catastrophic reaction.

_____ 4. By knowing residents well and being aware of any of their misperceptions, staff can often avoid problem situations.

_____ 5. A suspicious resident often hears very well and thus knows that people are saying bad things about the resident.

_____ 6. Abusive residents may be more cooperative if allowed to make some choices and have some control over their lives.

_____ 7. A friendly touch on the arm or hand of lonely persons will only make them feel worse.

_____ 8. Major tranquilizers are rarely effective in controlling agitation and aggression.

_____ 9. There is no point to understanding reasons for residents' problem behavior, as this won't help solve the problem.

_____ 10. Sleeping pills are effective in bringing on sleep in the elderly but should only be used on a short-term basis.

REFERENCES

Allen-Burge, R., Stevens, A. B., & Burgio, L. D. (1999). Effective behavioral interventions for decreasing dementia-related challenging behavior in nursing homes. *International Journal of Geriatric Psychiatry, 14,* 213–232.

Anonymous. (1998, April). Treatment of agitation in older persons with dementia. *Postgraduate Medicine,* pp. 1–88.

Aronson, M. K. (1983). The acting-out elderly: An overview. In M. K. Aronson, R. Bennett, & B. J. Gurland (Eds.), *The acting-out elderly* (pp. 3–13). New York: Haworth Press.

Astrom, S., Nilsson, M., Norberg, A., & Winblad, B. (1990). Empathy, experience of burnout and attitudes towards demented patients among nursing staff in geriatric care. *Journal of Advanced Nursing, 15,* 1236–1244.

Barnes, R., et al. (1982). Efficacy of antipsychotic medications in behaviorally disturbed dementia patients. *American Journal of Psychiatry, 139,* 1170–1174.

Bernabei, R., Gambassi, G., Lapane, K., Sgadari, A., Landi, F., Gatsonis, C., Lipsitz, L., & Mor, V. (1999). Characteristics of the SAGE database: A new resource for research on outcomes in long-term care. SAGE (Systematic Assessment of Geriatric drug use via Epidemiology) Study Group. *Journals of Gerontology, Series A, Biological Sciences & Medical Sciences, 54*(1), M25–M33.

Bernier, S. L., & Small, N. R. (1988). Disruptive behaviors. *Journal of Gerontological Nursing, 14*(2), 8–13.

Burgio, L. D., et al. (1988). Behavior problems in an urban nursing home. *Journal of Gerontological Nursing, 14*(1), 31–34.

Clinton, M., Moyle, W., Weir, D., & Edwards, H. (1995). Perceptions of stressors and reported coping strategies in nurses caring for residents with

---

Answers: 1-T, 2-T, 3-T, 4-T, 5-F, 6-T, 7-F, 8-F, 9-F, 10-T.

Alzheimer's disease in a dementia unit. *Australian & New Zealand Journal of Mental Health Nursing, 4*(1), 5–13.

Cohen, C. A., & Pushkar, D. (1999). Transitions in care: Lessons learned from a longitudinal study of dementia care. *American Journal of Geriatric Psychiatry, 7,* 139–146.

Cohen-Mansfield, J. (1999). Measurement of inappropriate behavior associated with dementia. *Journal of Gerontological Nursing, 25*(2), 42–51.

Cohen-Mansfield, J., Marx, M. S., & Rosenthal, A. S. (1989). A description of agitation in a nursing home. *Journal of Gerontology, 44*(3), M77–84.

Cox, R. A. (1998). Implementing nurse sensitive outcomes into care planning at a long-term-care facility. *Journal of Nursing Care Quality, 12*(5), 41–51.

Cummings, J. L., et al. (1987). Neuropsychiatric aspects of multi-infarct dementia and dementia of the Alzheimer type. *Archives of Neurology, 44,* 389–393.

Davis, L. L., Buckwalter, K., & Burgio, L. D. (1997). Measuring problem behaviors in dementia: Developing a methodological agenda. *Advances in Nursing Science, 20*(1), 40–55.

Gwyther, L. P. (1985). *Care of Alzheimer's patients: A manual for nursing home staff.* Chicago: American Health Care Association and Alzheimer's Disease and Related Disorders Association.

Hansebo, G., Kihlgren, M., Ljunggren, G., & Winblad, B. (1998). Staff views on the resident assessment instrument, RAI/MDS, in nursing homes, and the use of the cognitive performance scale, CPS, in different levels of care in Stockholm, Sweden. *Journal of Advanced Nursing, 28,* 642–653.

Jenike, M. A. (1989). *Geriatric psychiatry and psychopharmacology: A clinical approach.* Chicago: Yearbook Medical Publishers.

Jones, M. K. (1985). Patient violence. *Journal of Psychosocial Nursing, 23*(6), 12–17.

Lawton, M. P., Casten, R., Parmelee, P. A., Van Haitsma, K., Corn, J., & Kleban, M. H. (1998). Psychometric characteristics of the minimum data set II: Validity. *Journal of the American Geriatrics Society, 46*(6), 736–744.

Lehninger, F. W., Ravindran, V. L., & Stewart, J. T. (1998). Management strategies for problem behavior in the patient with dementia. *Geriatrics, 53*(4), 55–56, 66–68, 71–75.

Mace, N., & Rabins, P. (1981). *The 36-hour day.* Baltimore, MD: John Hopkins University Press.

Morrant, J. C., & Ablog, J. R. (1983). The angry elderly patient. *Postgraduate Medicine, 74*(6), 93–102.

Ouslander, J. G., Osterweil, D., & Morley, J. (1997). *Medical care in the nursing home* (2nd ed.). New York: McGraw-Hill.

Raskind, M. A., Risse, S. C., & Lampe, T. H. (1987). Dementia and antipsychotic drugs. *Journal of Clinical Psychiatry, 48,* 16–18.

Reisberg, B., et al. (1987). Behavioral symptoms in Alzheimer's disease: Phenomenology and treatment. *Journal of Clinical Psychiatry, 48,* 9–15.

Ryden, M. B. (1989). *Behavioral problems in dementia: A review of the literature.* Proceedings from the First Conference on Nursing Research and Clinical Management of Alzheimer's Disease. Minneapolis, MN: University of Minnesota.

Salzman, C. (1987). Treatment of the elderly agitated patient. *Journal of Clinical Psychiatry, 48,* 19–22.

Schweiger, J. L., & Huey, R. A. (1999). Alzheimer's disease: Your role in the caregiving equation. *Nursing, 99,* 35–41.

Sherman, D. S. (1988, November). Use of psychoactive drugs for the behaviorally disturbed. *Provider,* pp. 32–36.

Tappen, R. (1997). *Intervention for Alzheimer's disease: A caregiver's complete reference.* Baltimore, MD: Health Professions.

Thomas, D. R. (1988). Assessment and management of agitation in the elderly. *Geriatrics, 43*(6), 45–53.

Watson, R., Modeste, N. N., Catolico, O., & Crouch, M. (1998). The relationship between caregiver burden and self-care deficits in former rehabilitation patients. *Rehabilitation Nursing, 23,* 258–262.

Winger, J., Schirm, V., & Stewart, D. (1987). Aggressive behavior in long term care. *Journal of Psychosocial Nursing and Mental Health Services, 25,* 28–33.

Winograd, C. H., & Jarvik, L. F. (1986). Physician management of the demented patient. *Journal of the American Geriatrics Society, 34,* 295–308.

Winogrond, I. R. (Ed.). (1984, April). *Intervention and treatment of paranoia in older community residents.* Paper presented at seminar of the Long-term Care Gerontological Center of Milwaukee.

Zarit, S. H. (1996). Interventions with family caregivers. In S. H. Zarit & B. G. Knight (Eds.), *A guide to psychotherapy and aging: Effective clinical interventions in a life-stage context* (pp. 139–158). Washington, DC: American Psychological Association.

Zarit, S. H., Orr, N. K., & Zarit, J. M. (1985). *The hidden victims of Alzheimer's disease.* New York: New York University Press.

Zimmer, J. G., Watson, N., & Treat, A. (1984). Behavioral problems among patients in skilled nursing facilities. *American Journal of Public Health, 74,* 1118–1121.

Feeding Strategies

LEARNING OBJECTIVES

- To recognize the importance of food and eating in a high-quality life
- To use feeding strategies that promote good food intake
- To use different techniques at each stage of dementia
- To recognize the problems with feeding tubes and how to address them

PRETEST

Place a "T" before true statements, an "F" before false statements, and a question mark before those you don't know.

_____ 1. Food is important to a demented person.

_____ 2. Professional staff are usually well trained in feeding techniques.

_____ 3. Nursing home residents are typically overweight.

_____ 4. Because feeding residents is so important, nursing homes hire enough staff to accomplish this task.

_____ 5. Residents often feel thirsty.

_____ 6. Having the television on while feeding encourages residents to eat more.

＿＿ 7. Residents should be fed while they are in a seated position.
＿＿ 8. Thickener is often added to the food and liquids of a severely demented person.
＿＿ 9. Demented residents can usually be fed in 10 minutes.
＿＿ 10. Demented residents need encouragement while they are eating.

Food is an integral part of a high-quality life. Eating may be the last pleasure for some older adults. Sadly, for elders with dementia, selecting favorite foods, eating on their own, and even swallowing may be abilities they are losing as their disease progresses. Given the losses faced by older adults with dementia, it is critically important for us to help preserve the abilities and choices they do have. Feeding is one key to the happiness of a demented elder.

What does it feel like to be fed? We may have vague memories of our own childhood, where we were fed by mothers encouraging us to "open the garage door." We may remember the choo-choo spoon steaming toward a reluctant mouth. We also treasure that feeling of being loved as we were fed. We may have pictures of ourselves covered in food and smiles. We may have delighted in squishing peas, carefully picking up Cheerios, smearing our face with chocolate ice cream, turning tongues and lips blue with popsicles.

Where did we learn how to feed our children? As parents, no one really showed us how. The Lamaze class didn't prepare us for this. We bought the formula, panicking at the directions. Soon we were pros. We bought the jars of baby food, the small spoons covered in plastic, the bibs. For hungry babies and toddlers, feeding was easy. However, the picky eaters were the real challenge, calling on our imaginations for train imagery, coaxing, and special foods.

Health care schools devote very little of their curricula to this most important skill. It is thought to be so simple and easy that almost anyone can do it. And so we develop our own techniques, assuring ourselves that we are getting the job done.

However, many nursing home residents lose weight (Ouslander, Osterweil, & Morley, 1997; Sanders, Hoffman, & Lund, 1992). Residents aspirate food, some dying of aspiration pneumonia. Staff complain of not enough help to feed their patients—they rush through

---

Answers: 1-T, 2-F, 3-F, 4-F, 5-F, 6-F, 7-T, 8-T, 9-F, 10-T.

feeding, feed several patients as if in an assembly line, sometimes overlook feeding patients, or feed only partial meals. Residents get agitated during meals, may refuse to eat, or may fall asleep during meals.

Competently feeding a demented resident is a complicated and intertwined exchange between the feeder and eater (Van Ort & Phillips, 1992). Van Ort and Phillips (1992) taped 29 different feeding sessions. They found a disorganized series of events that showed much need for training in the feeder staff they observed.

GENERAL FEEDING GUIDELINES

An assessment of the resident's preferences and mealtime patterns is the initial task of anyone providing feeding assistance. Hellen (1998) suggests the use of the LifeStory to elicit this information. The Life-Story is a resident book filled with information about a person's key life events, work history, family background, recreational interests, favorite holidays, favorite foods and recipes, and other important historical facts pertaining to the person. Residents must be continually reassessed as their cognitive abilities and physical health change.

Adequate nutrition and hydration are critical for good health. A resident should have a well-balanced diet and plenty of fluids. Adequate protein is particularly important in the healing of pressure ulcers. Fiber and fluids are critical to prevent constipation. Dehydration can also cause delirium in addition to the cognitive impairment of dementia.

Hellen (1998) encourages multisensory cueing during feeding— using all of the resident's senses to encourage food intake. The appearance, aromas, flavors, and textures of food should be pleasing to the resident. Allow delicious food smells to permeate the dining area—the smell of popcorn, baking bread or cookies, cinnamon, and perking coffee get digestive juices flowing. The staff person feeding the resident should also describe what the resident is going to be eating, for example, "Here comes a spoonful of mashed potatoes" or "This chocolate pudding looks delicious."

Foods should be well prepared. Hot foods should be hot, cold foods cold. They should be tempting to the resident, and when possible, be ethnically preferred foods.

Feed in a quiet, comfortable environment. Make sure the eating area looks like a dining room. Turn off TVs and radios. Simplify the appearance of the tray. Residents may be confused by too many foods or utensils. Make sure that the food is a contrasting color to the plate. Residents may overlook white potatoes on a white plate. Observe what the resident is actually eating; sometimes residents try to eat napkins or other nonfood items, mistaking them for food. They may also get more food on themselves than in themselves.

Make sure the resident is up and ready to be fed. The resident should be groomed in preparation for feeding, with eyeglasses put on, hearing aid in, and dentures in place. If at all possible, the resident should be seated in a chair.

Take adequate time to feed. Feeding a demented resident his or her entire meal may take as much as an hour or even longer. If the resident wants to feed himself or herself at times during the meal, permit this. Residents may reach for finger foods and eat on their own. Be aware of which time of day your resident prefers eating. Some of us never eat breakfast, whereas others enjoy a hearty breakfast. Notice individual preferences in your residents.

Before the meal is even offered to a resident, make preparations. Get plenty of towels or napkins. Make sure utensils are small enough, as some residents have trouble opening their mouths wide. Make sure plenty of thickener is on hand. Some dietary departments provide several small packets of thickener on the tray. This is rarely enough. Have a large container of thickener nearby. Puddings, gelatin, and melted ice cream work well as thickeners in milk. Thickening agents themselves often clump up or turn into a hard, rock-like consistency without adequate stirring. Thickener must be stirred for a long time in milk. Jello may be added to water to make it thicker for residents with swallowing difficulties. Plastic cups may need a section cut out to make room for the resident's nose.

Some residents may not be able to communicate verbally that they are hungry or may not recognize that they are hungry. Others may not feel hungry because of decreased activity or side effects of medication. Medications may cause dry mouth, which interferes with chewing and digestive ability. Other drugs may cause tremors or other Parkinson-like symptoms, making the holding of utensils difficult for self-feeding.

Some residents need extra calories. Make sure to put butter on bread and vegetables. Always use condiments to make food more palatable to the resident; add salt and pepper appropriately. Residents may enjoy sweet foods. Add sugar to coffee and tea if they prefer sweet drinks. Sometimes adding sugar or fruit juice to food may make it more enticing to a particular resident.

Set the resident up in as much of a 90-degree angle as possible. Food goes down the esophagus more easily if the resident is sitting upright. Use cushions and special chairs provided by the Occupational Therapy department to get the resident in the correct position. Consult with speech pathology about the best head position for the resident. Some residents need a head down position. Some need to turn to one side or the other if they have had a stroke. Find out if stroking the resident's neck is a good idea to encourage swallowing.

Provide plenty of social interaction and coaxing during mealtime. Some elders need positive reinforcement after every bite. They may need to hear, "That's good."

Mr. Pfeiffer would smile and coo when praised during eating. He would eat much more of his meal if his feeder encouraged him and praised him after every mouthful.

Some need encouragement to actually open their mouths and swallow the bite of food. You can mirror the required action by opening your own mouth.

The same caregiver should feed the resident whenever possible. Thirty different staff members fed a resident during a 1-month period in a study conducted in Sweden (Backstrom, Norberg, & Norberg, 1987). Residents will often eat better for a certain caregiver.

When his LPN was transferred to a different floor, Mr. Johnson refused to eat. Ms. Garcia had to be loaned to her prior unit during mealtime so that Mr. Johnson could be coaxed into eating.

Be aware of how much the resident is actually eating and drinking The resident may seem more functional than he or she actually is. It is better to provide assistance than ignore the resident. Kayser-Jones and Schell (1997) suggest that labeling a resident as "difficult" gives staff implicit permission to ignore the resident. A resident may be extremely hungry but lack the communication ability to tell you this. Observe the resident and make sure that he or she is truly able to get food into the mouth and adequately chew and swallow.

Be educated about resident choking. If the airway is completely blocked, immediately perform a Heimlich maneuver or get assistance from a trained staff member.

The following recommendations are for feeding mildly demented elders, moderately demented elders, and severely demented elders.

FEEDING STRATEGIES FOR MILD DEMENTIA

Mildly demented elders need some help with mealtime. They may have apraxia, which is difficulty in carrying out intentional physical activities. Therefore, they may have trouble in opening milk cartons, getting straws out of the white paper covering, or adding condiments appropriately. They may need some beginning assistance in using utensils, but once started, may continue well on their own. They may need adaptive equipment, which is usually provided through an occupational-therapy consultation.

Mildly demented elders may also be feeling depressed or anxious. Depressed elders may want to skip eating, or eat more for comfort. Anxious persons may want to cope with anxiety through comfort foods, candy, alcohol, or physical activity. Caregivers should provide comfort foods, but make sure that nutritious foods are also being eaten.

Mildly demented elders may experience paranoia. They may think that family or staff are out to get them or even poison them.

Miss Phillips would only eat foods that came prepackaged.

Medications should not be mixed into the foods of paranoid residents.

Caffeine may need to be eliminated in agitated residents. Caffeine withdrawal may cause a severe headache, so withdraw residents gradually.

Even in the mild stage, elders with dementia may forget foods they recently consumed. They should not be questioned about what they ate at a particular meal. Caregivers should monitor the tray carefully to see what is actually being eaten. Residents may want to eat off the trays of others. Try to discourage this, as residents may have some dietary limitations such as low sodium or a diabetic diet.

Older adults often do not feel thirsty. Caregivers at this stage should make an effort to provide plenty of fluids and encourage drinking. Fluids should be encouraged throughout the day.

As mildly demented elders become increasingly demented, they may get more food on them than in them when they eat. Caregivers should be alert to the changing stage and provide more assistance to the resident. Smaller, simpler meals may become more enticing to the resident. Offer supplements, juices, water, and snacks throughout the day as staffing permits.

FEEDING STRATEGIES FOR MODERATE DEMENTIA

This is the most problematic stage for feeding. Some patients will want to wander continuously, making a sit-down meal difficult to accomplish. They need finger foods and midmeal supplements. Wanderers need more calories because of their constant exercise, but caregivers often feel frustrated as to how to provide these foods. Perhaps a small hip purse filled with nutritious finger foods will solve this problem (Hellen, 1998). Foods need to be nutrient dense.

Some residents may refuse food. They will turn their heads, keep their mouths shut, spit out food, or push the feeder's spoon away (Volicer et al., 1989). Why don't they want to eat? They may not be hungry because of little or no activity during the day. They may not recognize their hunger. They may be frightened by choking. They may be depressed. They may not want to eat the type of food being served. It may be quite painful for them to open their mouths, chew, or swallow. A dental appointment to assess teeth is important for the resident who seems to find chewing painful. A speech pathologist can determine if esophagus problems may be causing pain.

Some persons will be hyperoral. Everything goes into the mouth, including many nonfood items such as tacks or styrofoam bits. These items are a choking, poison, and laceration danger. A resident may try to eat a napkin. Chemicals on housekeeping carts are a particular danger. Plants may also be poisonous, so only safe plants should be inside the unit or in the wandering area.

Some residents will hoard food. They will keep a bite in their cheek or pocket for hours on end. Residents may hide food in drawers. Staff must be vigilant about cleaning out drawers, or bugs may become a problem. Cheeks need to be checked for food, and brushing of teeth must be encouraged or carried out for the resident.

Residents may tire during the meal and consume only a portion of it.

Mr. Johnson, who also had Parkinson's disease as well as dementia, would fall asleep several times during a meal. He had to be gently awakened.

Some residents may become easily agitated by television left on during the meal. TVs and radios should be turned off, and other noise should be silenced during mealtime.

FEEDING STRATEGIES FOR SEVERE DEMENTIA

As dementia progresses, swallowing ability should be routinely assessed by the speech pathologist. Swallowing may become difficult for demented persons, or they may forget to swallow. The demented person may aspirate food particles and liquids into airways and are then at risk for developing aspiration pneumonia. The speech pathologist may conduct a bedside evaluation or recommend a radiographic study. During such a procedure, the older adult swallows liquids or solids mixed with barium while being x-rayed, and the specialist studies the path of the bolus of liquid or food. The speech pathologist will recommend a special consistency of food and liquids if there is a problem. Certain postures and positions of the head and neck will also be recommended. The head-down position is often an easier position in which to swallow food. This has implications for feeders. Feeders cannot stand above the resident when feeding; they must sit at eye level.

To assist swallowing, foods are often chopped up finely (a mechanical diet) or pureed. Liquids must be thickened with a thickening product, pudding, or melted ice cream.

Don't mix foods together unnecessarily. Mashed potatoes can usually be added to meat for thickening. However, respect the separate flavors of foods whenever possible.

If the risk of aspiration is too great, physicians may recommend a feeding tube. This tube is surgically placed in the stomach. Liquids are poured through the tube at specified times. Some products are fed continuously to the resident if the person is seriously underweight. The benefits of a tube are the provision of adequate nutrition and lessening of staff time to feed the patient. The down side is that residents must give up one of their greatest pleasures—eating. Residents may also be tempted to pull out tubes, which may cause the facility to institute restraints. Volicer and colleagues (1989) suggest that some feeding tubes do not prevent aspiration, can cause restriction in activity, and deprive the resident of the pleasures of eating and staff contact. Volicer et al. (1990) encourage tube feeding be replaced by natural feeding for most AD patients.

The pros and cons of feeding tubes are important concerns to the patient, family, and entire medical team. It is recommended that such decisions go before a nursing home ethics committee before feeding-tube placement.

SUMMARY

Eating is one of the last pleasures of a demented older adult. Feeding demented residents is a challenging task. At various stages in dementia, there are a variety of difficult problems related to eating and feeding. Staff must be thoroughly trained in proper feeding techniques. An interdisciplinary effort of several disciplines is required to make feeding a safe, pleasurable experience for the resident.

LEARNING EXERCISES

1. Get a tray of food from the dietary department. Have a colleague feed it to you. How does this make you feel?
2. With a tray of pureed food, eat one bite from each item. How does it taste? Then, mix several of the food items together. Sample the mixture. How does it taste?
3. Observe several nursing home staff while they feed their residents. Notice the techniques that seem to help residents eat more. List five of these techniques.
4. If you are not assigned to feed residents, volunteer to feed a resident once a week.
5. Try praising a severely demented resident after each mouthful of food. Notice the effect of this encouragement.
6. Make a special effort to get a resident who usually eats in bed cleaned and up in a chair before a meal. Be sure to put on the resident's glasses, dentures, and hearing aid. Then notice whether your resident is eating better.
7. Before the next meal, turn off all TVs, radios, and alarms in the environment. Chat quietly with the resident during the meal. Evaluate the impact of this on resident agitation and food intake.

8. List all residents or patients in your facility who are tube fed. Discuss with the health care team the possibility of returning these patients to natural feeding.

POSTTEST

Put a "T" before true statements, an "F" before false statements, and a question mark before those you don't know.

_____ 1. Many nursing home residents lose weight.
_____ 2. Feeding a resident is often a disorganized experience.
_____ 3. An assessment of the resident's preferences and mealtime patterns can be conducted with the help of the LifeStory.
_____ 4. Dehydration can cause delirium.
_____ 5. Feeding a demented resident may take an hour or longer.
_____ 6. Thickener will often cause aspiration.
_____ 7. Salt, pepper, and sugar should not be added to the foods of demented residents.
_____ 8. Use many different caregivers to feed a demented resident.
_____ 9. It is important to mix pureed foods together.
_____ 10. Feeding tubes may be pulled out by a demented resident.

REFERENCES

Backstrom, A., Norberg, A., & Norberg, B. (1987). Feeding difficulties in long stay patients at nursing homes. *International Journal of Nursing Studies, 24,* 69–76.

Hellen, C. R. (1998). Eating: Mealtime challenges and interventions. In M. Kaplan & S. B. Hoffman (Eds.), *Behaviors in dementia: Best practices for successful management* (pp. 193–226). Baltimore, MD: Health Professions Press.

Kayser-Jones, J., & Schell, E. (1997). The mealtime experience of a cognitively impaired elder: Ineffective and effective strategies. *Journal of Gerontological Nursing, 23*(7), 33–39.

Ouslander, J. G., Osterweil, D., & Morley, J. (Eds.). (1997). *Medical care in the nursing home* (pp. 187–202). New York: McGraw-Hill.

Answers: 1-T, 2-T, 3-T, 4-T, 5-T, 6-F, 7-F, 8-F, 9-F, 10-T.

Sanders, H. N., Hoffman, S. B., & Lund, C. (1992). Feeding strategies for dependent eaters. *Journal of the American Medical Association, 2,* 1389–1390.

Van Ort, S., & Phillips, L. (1992). Feeding nursing home residents with Alzheimer's disease. *Geriatric Nursing, 13,* 249–253.

Volicer, L., Seltzer, B., Rheaume, Y., Karner, J., Glennon, M., Riley, M. E., & Crino, P. (1989). Eating difficulties in patients with probable dementia of the Alzheimer type. *Journal of Geriatric Psychiatry and Neurology, 2,* 188–195.

Volicer, L., Rheaume, Y., Riley, M. E., Karner, J., & Glennon, M. (1990). Discontinuation of tube feeding in patients with dementia of the Alzheimer type. *American Journal of Alzheimer's Care and Related Disorders and Research, 5,* 22–25.

Wandering

LEARNING OBJECTIVES

- To identify the deficits and behaviors that are associated with wandering
- To learn how to analyze different types of wandering
- To discover possible causes for wandering
- To learn how to intervene to decrease wandering
- To minimize the problems arising from wandering

PRETEST

Place a "T" before true statements, an "F" before false statements, and a question mark before those you don't know.

_____ 1. Only severely demented persons wander.
_____ 2. A person who feels lost may wander to try to find a familiar place.
_____ 3. Some persons who seem to pace aimlessly really are doing it for exercise.
_____ 4. A disoriented person who has to use the bathroom may start wandering.
_____ 5. Persons who are in pain usually sit quietly so as to keep from hurting more.

_____ 6. A cognitively impaired person who has always coped with stress with physical activity is more likely to turn to wandering when stressed.

_____ 7. Providing activities for wanderers only increases their wandering.

_____ 8. When retrieving someone who has wandered away from the facility, the caregiver should stand in front of the person, making the person turn around and head back.

_____ 9. Only nursing staff needs to know about the facility's policies and approaches to wandering behavior and which residents are more likely to wander.

_____ 10. Placing some interesting objects to touch near an exit may distract wanderers sufficiently so that they don't try to leave.

Wandering is a serious problem to those who care for the confused or cognitively impaired older person. In fact, a survey of administrators and nursing personnel in long-term-care facilities indicated that resident wandering was their leading behavioral problem (Branzelle, 1988); moreover, the incidence of wandering among nursing home residents ranges from 11% to 38% (Algase, 1992; Rovner, Kafonek, Filipp, Lucas, & Folstein, 1986; U.S. Department of Health & Human Services, 1989 as cited in Holmberg, 1997a). Wandering is listed as one of the three most common behaviors cited for transferring patients from nursing homes to state mental hospital (Moak & Fisher, 1990 as cited in Holmberg, 1997a). Wandering refers to the tendency of a person who is cognitively impaired (Algase, Kupferschmid, Beel-Bates, & Beattie, 1997) to move about an area in an apparently aimless fashion (Snyder et al., 1978). Wandering may also involve a person trying to get to some specific, often unobtainable place such as a childhood home that no longer exists.

Mrs. Woods walks in and out of the door to the garden area of her dementia-specific unit, continually asking staff if they can help her get to her home in Scranton.

Although people who wander may appear to have cognitive deficits, a person with little or no dementia can also engage in wandering

Answers: 1-F, 2-T, 3-T, 4-T, 5-F, 6-T, 7-F, 8-F, 9-F, 10-T.

behavior; Algase et al. (1997) assert that wandering is a phenomenon displayed to some extent by all independently ambulatory, cognitively intact nursing home residents. Usually such an individual can give an easily understandable reason for the behavior, such as wanting exercise. Also, because such persons usually have better judgment, they cause fewer problems for caregivers.

WHY WANDERING IS A PROBLEM

Wandering presents a problem to the caregiver in three major areas. The first problem is safety. A person who is wandering will often leave the building through the first door seen. Especially in cases of severe cognitive impairment, the wanderer may not be able to appreciate such common dangers as busy streets, frigid weather, loss of sense of direction, and so on. The person often quickly becomes lost, even in a familiar neighborhood.

> *Mr. Alessi left the house to go for a newspaper at the neighborhood store. He apparently turned the corner a block too soon and was found several hours later on the street behind his house, totally lost. Being lost, the wanderer became frightened, which further reduces his ability to cope. This can be a very dangerous situation.*

We have all heard of incidents in which an older person wandered away from his residence and was not found for several days, often too late to save him. To the caregiver who has responsibility for the welfare of the resident, this is certainly the most frightening consequence of wandering. But even other less serious outcomes to wandering are stressful to caregivers. The anxiety of the family and caregiver, the bewilderment of the wanderer who feels lost, and a search and rescue by the police are all stresses that are experienced when a wanderer gets lost.

The second area in which wandering causes a problem is with interpersonal relations. The wanderer, in the course of wandering around a facility, can severely strain the patience and goodwill of fellow residents.

> *Mrs. Abbott daily walks in and out of the rooms of several residents on the first floor, without an invitation to enter. She often claims that the room and contents are her own, much to the upset of the rightful owner. Staff are often*

called on to restore peace in such situations, reaffirm the property rights of the
rightful owner, and guide the wanderer back to neutral territory.

As part of a study on disruptive behavior (Bernier & Small, 1988), residents in a nursing home were asked to rate resident behaviors that they found most disruptive to their living environment. Residents rated other residents entering the wrong room as the most disruptive behavior out of 22 possible disruptive behaviors. Residents of long-term-care facilities can become extremely angry about a person who habitually wanders into their room. It takes a lot of staff time to intercede, smooth ruffled feelings, and try to prevent further incidents.

The third area in which wandering presents a problem is in the area of health. In some cases a person who wanders is in frail physical health and can wander to the point of damaging health.

Mr. Arbor is an example of a wanderer who walks so much that he developed
open sores on his feet. He would walk about 8 hours a day, and even the softest
shoes would not prevent him from developing blisters and raw red areas on
his heels, toes, and bottom of this feet.

Wanderers have been known to keep moving to the point of exhaustion, worsening cardiac problems or other chronic ailments. Although we know that mild to moderate exercise can be very healthful, excessive participation in any activity can cause problems.

WHY PEOPLE WANDER

What causes a person to wander? Several reasons have been identified. Some people have throughout their lives responded to stress with physical activity, for example, going for a walk to cool off after an argument. This pattern continues when they become cognitively impaired. Several research studies (Allen-Burge, Stevens, & Burgio, 1999; Monsour & Robb, 1982; Shoemaker, 1987; Snyder et al., 1978) have cited the connection between previous lifestyle or coping mechanisms and later wandering behavior. It is suggested that intake interviews in long-term-care facilities include a discussion of previous activities, coping styles, and ways of handling stress (Monsour & Robb, 1982). This information could be used to predict wandering behavior and provide ideas for managing such behavior if it occurs.

A related cause of wandering behavior is the feeling of restlessness, anxiety, or agitation, which produces the need for some activity. The only activity available may be walking back and forth in the halls. Physical symptoms are another cause of wandering. Many demented people start wandering either because they sense the need to use the toilet or because they have been incontinent. The inability to communicate needs or desires, (i.e., hunger, not knowing where to find the toilet) can cause "search" behaviors (Holmberg, 1997a), which lead them to wander around looking for an appropriate place to meet their needs.

Pain can sometimes cause a person to wander.

When Mrs. Largo was experiencing pain from a hiatal hernia, she would walk up and down the hall repeatedly saying, "Oh dear, how do I get out of here? I'm so sick."

Also, certain medications, even tranquilizers, may cause a feeling of restlessness that results in increased wandering.

Another cause of wandering may be tension or stress in the environment. Caregivers in long-term-care facilities often note an increase in wandering behavior when things are particularly hectic on a unit, such as a change of shift (Hiatt, 1980; Snyder et al., 1978). Wandering residents seem to respond to increased activity of the staff with their own increase in activity.

Nighttime wandering can be a truly severe problem, especially for the caregiver in the home who badly needs a good night's sleep (Young et al., 1988). Nighttime wanderers are often disoriented to time. They usually have had their sleep and wake cycle disrupted and are unaware that it is time to sleep. In addition, it can be stressful to be awake at night when many of the orienting cues of daytime—light, sounds, and people—are out of sight. Wandering at night can be a way of alleviating stress for the resident, who may be searching for cues to get a better understanding of the surroundings.

The primary characteristic of most people who wander is memory impairment and disorientation. The person may have set out with some goal in mind, made a wrong turn into unfamiliar territory, and kept wandering around, trying to get back. This may especially happen when a person is moved to a new environment. A person who is "living in the past" may be caught up in a schedule maintained years ago. Such a person feels a great need to get somewhere—to work, home to fix supper for the children, home to mother who will be worried because the person is missing (Monsour & Robb, 1982; Rader, 1987; Snyder et al., 1978). This need to be somewhere else can be quite desperate. Dealing with it requires all the ingenuity the caregiver has.

Mr. Greene jumps out of bed every morning at 6:00 and dresses himself in a three-piece suit, which his family has brought in for him. He looks over a copy of the paper in the dining room, even though he can no longer understand it. Then Mr. Greene says to the staff, "Where do I go to get the 7:45 bus? I can't be late to work today—important appointment." A staff member chats with him, asking him questions about his work and acknowledging his pride in good attendance and punctuality. She then indicates to Mr. Greene that today is a holiday from work and that he can have the whole day off to relax and enjoy his hobbies. He soon gets involved in recreational therapy and craft activities of the nursing home, which he enjoys. Because of his memory impairment, he appears unaware that every day is now a holiday for him.

TYPES OF WANDERING BEHAVIOR

Wandering has been systematically studied in long-term-care facilities in an effort to understand it and find better ways to control it. One study (Snyder et al., 1978) identifies four types of wandering behavior differentiated by energy level and whether or not there was a defined goal (see Table 8.1). The first type is described by a high energy level and a clearly observable goal, for example, the person intends to go "home" or some other designated place—as in the wandering of Mr. Greene. A second type shows a high energy level but apparently has no defined goal. The activity itself is the object of the wandering. Wanderers of this type often seem to be busy "puttering around" as they move from place to place. They apparently find the movement soothing. A third type has a low energy level but has a defined goal firmly held in mind. This type waits quietly in a strategic spot, and when the opportunity presents itself, the person, like Houdini, unexpectedly and successfully wanders away from the facility.

One 85-year-old woman with moderately severe dementia quietly left her boarding home one morning and was found several blocks away at a school, asking for a job.

A fourth type of wanderer shows a low energy level and no defined goal. A "pacer" who moves slowly with little apparent direction is an example of this type.

TABLE 8.1 Types of Wandering

Type/description	Suggestions for management
High energy level—goal directed, wants "out," wants to "go home."	1. Provide exercise. 2. Supervise in outside activities. 3. Restraints probably won't work.
High energy level—no defined goal, activity itself is the goal, "industrious putterer," movement is soothing.	1. Involve in simple repetitive diversional activities. 2. Ask: Is this really a problem?
Low energy level—goal directed "Houdini," who unexpectedly and successfully leaves facility.	1. Learn to anticipate conditions that lead to this behavior, and be prepared.
Low energy level—no defined goal, "pacer."	1. Check for environmental stimuli that may lead to agitation, e.g., noise, confusion. 2. Check for drug side effects or other physical problems such as pain. 3. Regular exercise programs may help.

Adapted from Snyder et al. (1978). Wandering. *Gerontologist, 18*, 272–280. Reprinted by permission of the publisher: The Gerontological Society of America.

By analyzing the type of wandering a person engages in, the caregiver can decide whether or not it is really a problem. Persons who appear to wander because they find the activity soothing, who stay within a defined, safe area, and who do not excessively interfere with other residents, probably should be allowed to pursue the activity.

For those whose wandering behavior does present a problem, caregivers can plan strategies and interventions that will be most effective for the type of wandering the person is engaging in. This will require a team effort with input, observations, and ideas from all levels of nursing staff and other disciplines.

MANAGING WANDERING BEHAVIORS

Wandering is a serious problem both for the caregiver in the home and caregiver in the long-term-care facility; a significant majority of persons with dementia receive care at home at considerable cost to their families (Aneshensel, Pearlin, & Schuler, 1993; Ingersoll-Dayton,

Starrels, & Dowler, 1996; Stommel, Given, Given, & Collins, 1995, as cited in Chang, 1999) and can create considerable stress for family members in their caregiving roles. Because there are several possible causes of wandering and a variety of ways in which wandering is expressed, the caregiver needs to know what to look for in the behavior, make some guesses as to why the resident is wandering, and plan the intervention on the basis of these observations.

Use of Restraints

The first thing often thought of when a resident presents a particularly serious and dangerous form of wandering behavior is to place the resident in a restraint of some sort. Some common restraints include geriatric wheelchairs (gerichairs) with a tray across the lap, and tie vests used while the person is in bed or in a chair. Although these methods may eliminate the behavior, the use of physical restraints has been associated with serious injuries and increased agitation (Cohen-Mansfield, Werner, Culpepper, & Barkley, 1997). Tranquilizing medications are also used as a form of chemical restraint. However, some medications can produce restlessness and wandering behavior as a side effect. This side effect is called "akathisia" and means an inability to sit still—just the opposite of what is intended (Thomas, 1988). At times it may be necessary to place a person who is persistently wandering in a dangerous fashion in a secure locked institution such as a mental hospital. Although such methods are usually effective in controlling the wandering and protecting the individual from harm, they are a serious infringement to the person's rights and freedom (Branzelle, 1988). Less drastic changes in the environment can provide some control over this behavior and better protect the person's rights.

Modifying the Physical Environment

Many persons who wander are demented and unable to learn how to operate devices with which they are unfamiliar. Thus, placing an unusual latch or locking device on a door or placing a latch or lock in an unconventional place on a door (e.g., at the top of the door above eye level or at the bottom of the door) may be enough to prevent a wanderer from getting out (Mace & Rabins, 1981). One facility actually had combination locks with the combination displayed prominently on the door. No wanderer was ever able to use that information to make an escape (Monsour & Robb, 1982).

Of course, for safety reasons many facilities are prohibited from maintaining locked doors. Some facilities have opted for buzzer systems that sound when an untended door is opened. However, a buzzer frequently going off can become quite annoying. Alternatively, the technology developed to thwart shoplifters can be used. The known wanderer can be provided with a bracelet or a belt that is continuously monitored by a scanner. If the scanner does not read the resident's signal, an alarm goes off that informs staff as to which resident is missing. Staff can locate the wanderer using a small unit to track the resident.

The problems of wandering can be helped by means of architecture and design. Because persons with dementia have a narrower range of cognitive coping, adjusting the physical and interpersonal environment is the most effective means to influence behavior (Ryden & Feldt, 1992 as cited in Holmberg, 1997a). Exit control and provision of the least-restrictive environment, which can help prevent elopement, can be difficult to achieve, but there are a number of ways to meet this goal (Tappen, 1997). A facility can be laid out in such a way that when you start walking in one direction, you eventually complete a circuit and return to the same place. This allows wanderers the freedom of wandering with little danger of getting lost. The same principle can be used outside in courtyards or in walkways that lead out one door and in another. Enclosed outdoor spaces can be planted with trees or shrubs in mazelike pathways to allow wanderers the impression they have had an unobstructed walk in an open space (Monsour & Robb, 1982). Doors to the outside can be subtly camouflaged with room dividers, mirrors, or other barriers (Coons, 1988; Fopma-Loy, 1988; Schafer, 1985); use of a cloth cover as a visual barrier for exit doors reduced exiting by 96% in a study by Dickinson, McLain-Kark, and Marshall-Baker (1995, as cited in Tappen, 1997). However, caution should be used whenever placing visual barriers on exits to assure safety concerns are met. One research study (Hussian & Brown, 1987) found that taping masking tape in a grid pattern on the floor about 3 feet from an exit door was successful in stopping seven out of eight demented wanderers from approaching the door. Placing a stop sign on the door can also be helpful. Wanderers can also be distracted from outside doors by establishing nearby an attractive place to sit down. Research has also shown that even highly active wanderers spend a good deal of their time sitting when they find a chair (Snyder et al., 1978). Some of their wandering might even be a search for a quiet, comfortable private place to sit down for a nap. Placing something of interest to manipulate near the door can also distract wanderers before they go out. One facility placed an "activity barrel" filled with plastic objects near an exit and found this attracted the attention of some wanderers, drawing their attention away from the door (Fopma-Loy, 1988; Gaffney, 1986).

Preparing the Social Environment

Another environmental approach to managing wandering is to ensure that the social environment of the facility and the neighborhood are as informed and protective as possible. Staff throughout the facility, including office workers, cleaners, and food service workers, should be informed and educated about wandering behavior and the facility policies and procedures for retrieving wanderers that have left the facility. Known wanderers should be introduced to staff and frequent visitors throughout the facility. This can be done in a friendly, unobtrusive way to protect the dignity of the wanderer but to allow others to know that the person is a resident of the facility and should be encouraged to remain there (Rader, 1987). Wanderers should have identification with them at all times. This is probably most easily accomplished by a wristband or bracelet imprinted with the pertinent information. It is also helpful for the band to have "memory impaired" written on it; this tactic should be suggested to family caregivers as few think of an ID band or bracelet unless it is suggested to them (Lach, Reed, Smith, & Carr, 1995 as cited in Tappen, 1997). Tappen (1997) notes that for a small fee, family caregivers can register their loved one with the Alzheimer's Association Safe Return Program, which offers an ID bracelet or necklace, wallet card, toll-free number to report when a loved one is lost, and guidance on the search process.

Just as staff members throughout the facility should be involved in the management of wandering behavior, so too persons in the neighborhood surrounding a long-term-care facility or private home can be enlisted to help. Contact can be made with the immediate neighbors, local shopkeepers, local police officers, and so on to inform them of the possibility of someone wandering away. You can inform them of what they should do if they encounter someone they believe has wandered away and thank them in advance for their interest and efforts. On some occasions, a facility might want to supply the local authorities with a photograph and identifying information about an individual who is particularly vulnerable to wandering away.

Retrieving a Wanderer

Once a person has left the living area or facility, how do you get the person back? Is it helpful to run after wandering individuals, grab them by the arm, and confront them with an angry voice and accusing looks? No, this is not the most effective way of retrieving a wanderer. In many cases, such an approach would lead to a catastrophic reaction and add to the caregiver's problems. A more effective approach is to quietly join the person. Walk along with the person in a friendly, calm manner, talking companionably about the day, where the person is going, and so on. After a short while, the caregiver can suggest something to change the direction of the walk, either sitting down for a moment or making a turn. With this approach, the wanderer can usually be led back with a minimum of trauma. This does take a certain amount of staff time and patience. It may not work for some single-minded "Houdini" types who know exactly where they are going and how to get there. But managing wandering escapades in this way protects the wanderer's dignity. It also helps develop trust in the caregiver and the facility and may cut down on the wanderer's feeling that there is an urgency to get away, thus reducing future wandering episodes (Gwyther, 1985; Rader, 1987; Snyder et al., 1978).

Active Interventions to Reduce Wandering

The management of wandering behavior can also be approached by understanding and dealing with the causes of the behavior. One must observe the wanderer, read the nonverbal message in the wandering, and try to understand why and under what circumstances the wandering occurs. Once there is some understanding of what causes wandering in a particular individual, intervention is possible. Is the person looking for a place to go to the toilet? Perhaps staff could establish a toileting regimen in which the resident is shown to the bathroom at regular intervals. Is the noise and confusion of a particularly busy time of day making the person restless? Perhaps the resident could be shown to a quiet, out-of-the-way place before activity begins. Does the quiet routine lead to boredom so that the person starts walking just for something to do? Structured, purposeful physical activities, such as a program of regular exercise to music or daily gardening hours, could be instituted to cut down on boredom.

Many facilities have introduced special programs to address the needs of persons who wander (McGrowder-Lin & Bhatt, 1988; Sawyer & Mendlovitz, 1982). One of the simplest programs to try is a regular routine of daily exercise. A programmed walking time, moving to music, simple calisthenics, ball toss, and parachute games are all possibilities for physical exercise most persons can participate in and enjoy. Walks outside, if at all possible, are particularly beneficial for restless wanderers. In a study by Holmberg (1997b), a walker's group was used as a successful nonpharmacologic clinical intervention for wandering; this is an activity that can be carried out by direct care staff or volunteers.

Sawyer and Mendlovitz (1982) reported on a program in one long-term-care facility in which the disruption caused by wanderers became a particularly serious problem. The wanderers were taken from the unit for 2 hours in the afternoon (a time when their behavior was especially disruptive on the unit) 4 days a week. They were taken to a special area that had access to an outside space and that could be secured so that they could safely wander. While there, they were involved in a special activity program. The structured program had five components: music, exercise, sensory stimulation, memory-recall or reminiscence, and nourishment. In addition, staff on the units received in-service education on coping techniques for managing wandering behaviors.

There were positive results for about half the participants in the program. The positive results included an increase in attention span, a decrease in incontinence, and a decrease in wandering and pillaging. Wanderers in the program began to spend time together outside the program, sitting side by side and chatting. In addition, the researchers noted a change in attitude toward the wanderers on the part of the staff. This change in attitude led to a reduction in the number of confrontations and a decrease in combativeness. All in all, this relatively simple program made a big impact on the problem of wandering at the facility.

SUMMARY

Wandering is and probably will always be a serious problem when caring for the cognitively impaired person, whether at home or in a long-term-care facility. But with some thought and ingenuity, it can be successfully managed. By observing the resident, deciding what type of wandering the person is engaging in, and the conditions under which the person wanders, effective intervention is achievable. Furthermore, caregivers should try to understand the residents needs, be flexible with providing personal care, maintain a calm environment, avoid physical and chemical restraints, use short concise words and sentences and use non-verbal cues (Cohen-Mansfield et al., 1997). The caregiver's goals are to preserve the rights and dignity of the individual who wanders, to protect other residents from intrusions into their living space, and to protect the wanderer from harmful situations.

LEARNING EXERCISES

1. Think of a time when you were really lost. Perhaps you were on your way to a wedding in a strange city. Or maybe it was the first day in a new school. Remember how it felt—the feeling that you were just going around in circles, the mounting fear you were going to be late, the panic that you would never find your way. Share some of your memories of such times with the group. Discuss what it might be like to be a disoriented wanderer who believes it is important to get somewhere.
2. In small groups, brainstorm different ways to manage wandering. Brainstorming means putting down every idea that comes up in the discussion without evaluating it. Then you can go through the list and select ideas that are possible to use and might be effective. Consider environmental changes, safety issues, activi-

ties that could be tried, and different staff approaches that could be used. Select the best ideas, and report back to the larger group.

3. One person plays the role of a wanderer who has successfully left the facility. Another person plays the role of a staff member trying to retrieve the wanderer. After role-playing this scene for 5 minutes, discuss the experience including what it felt like to be in these roles. Also, which strategies for bringing the wanderer back seemed ineffective and which strategies seemed most effective from the viewpoints of the wanderer, the retriever, and the audience?

POSTTEST

Place at "T" before true statements, an "F" before false statements, and a question mark before those you don't know.

_____ 1. Wearing an identification bracelet is of no use for a person who is apt to wander off.

_____ 2. The person who seems to be just puttering around and passing time when wandering might just as well be left alone as this rarely presents a problem to anyone.

_____ 3. Neighbors and local police should be contacted and given information about what they can do if they see a resident who appears to have wandered from the facility.

_____ 4. One of the most troubling things about some wanderers is their going into other residents' rooms uninvited.

_____ 5. Walks outside will probably just make most wanderers want to wander more.

_____ 6. Physical restraints are the only way to control wandering.

_____ 7. Some wanderers seem to want to get to a specific place, even though that place does not exist anymore.

_____ 8. A person's prior habits and way of life have little to do with wandering behavior.

_____ 9. Anxiety can be a cause for wandering, but boredom is not a cause.

_____ 10. Camouflaging a door to the outside sometimes can keep wanderers from using it to leave the facility.

Answers: 1-F, 2-T, 3-T, 4-T, 5-F, 6-F, 7-T, 8-F, 9-F, 10-T.

REFERENCES

Algase, D. L. (1992). A century of progress: Today's strategies for responding to wandering behavior. *Journal of Gerontological Nursing, 18*(11), 28–34.

Algase, D. L., Kupferschmid, B., Beel-Bates, C. A., & Beattie, E. R. A. (1997). Estimates of stability of daily wandering behavior among cognitively impaired long-term care residents. *Nursing Research, 46,* 172–178.

Allen-Burge, Stevens, & Burgio. (1999). Effective behavioral interventions for decreasing dementia-related challenging behavior in nursing homes. *International Journal of Geriatric Psychiatry, 14,* 213–232.

Aneshensel, C. S., Pearlin, L. I., & Schuler, R. H. (1993). Stress, role captivity, and the cessation of caregiving. *Journal of Health & Social Behavior, 34*(1), 54–70.

Bernier, S., & Small, N. R. (1988). Disruptive behaviors. *Journal of Gerontological Nursing, 14*(2), 8–13.

Branzelle, J. (1988, June). Provider responsibilities for care of wandering residents. *Provider,* pp. 22–23.

Chang, B. L. (1999). Cognitive-behavioral intervention for homebound caregivers of persons with dementia. *Nursing Research, 48,* 173–181.

Cohen-Mansfield, J., Werner, P., Culpepper, W. J., & Barkley, D. (1997). Evaluation of an inservice training program on dementia and wandering. *Journal of Gerontological Nursing, 23*(10), 40–47.

Coons, D. S. (1988). Wandering. *American Journal of Alzheimer's Care and Research, 3*(1), 31–36.

Fopma-Loy, J. (1988). Wandering: Causes, consequences and care. *Journal of Psychosocial Nursing and Mental Health Services, 26*(5), 8–18.

Gaffney, J. (1986). Toward a less restricted environment. *Geriatric Nursing, 7,* 94–95.

Gwyther, L. P. (1985). *Care of Alzheimer's patients: A manual for nursing home staff.* Chicago: Alzheimer's Disease and Related Disorders Association.

Hiatt, L. G. (1980, Mary/April). The happy wanderer. *Nursing Homes,* pp. 27–31.

Holmberg, S. K. (1997a). Evaluation of a clinical intervention for wanderers on a geriatric nursing unit. *Archives of Psychiatric Nursing, 11*(1), 21–28.

Holmberg, S. K. (1997b). A walking program for wanderers: Volunteer training and development of an evening walker's group. *Geriatric Nursing, 18,* 160–165.

Hussian, R. A., & Brown, D. C. (1987). Use of two-dimensional grid patterns to limit hazardous ambulation in demented patients. *Journal of Gerontology, 42,* 558–560.

Ingersoll-Dayton, B., Starrels, M. E., & Dowler, D. (1996). Caregiving for parents and parents-in-law: Is gender important? *Gerontologist, 36,* 483–491.

McGrowder-Lin, R., & Bhatt, A. (1988). A wanderer's lounge program for nursing home residents with Alzheimer's disease. *Gerontologist, 28*(5), 607–609.

Mace, N. L., & Rabins, R. (1981). *The 36-hour day: A family guide.* Baltimore, MD: John Hopkins University Press.

Monsour, N., & Robb, S. S. (1982). Wandering behavior in old age: A psychosocial study. *Social Work, 27,* 411–416.

Rader, J. (1987). A comprehensive staff approach to problem wandering. *Gerontologist, 27,* 756–760.

Rovner, B. W., Kafonek, S., Filipp, L., Lucas, M. J., & Folstein, M. F. (1986). Prevalence of mental illness in a community nursing home. *American Journal of Psychiatry, 143,* 1446–1449.

Sawyer, J. C., & Mendlovitz, A. (1982, November). *A management program for ambulatory institutionalized patients with Alzheimer's disease and related disorders.* Paper presented at Annual Gerontological Society of America Conference, Boston.

Schafer, S. (1985). Modifying the environment. *Geriatric Nursing, 6,* 157–159.

Shoemaker, D. (1987). Problematic behavior and the Alzheimer patient: Retrospection as a method of understanding and counseling. *Gerontologist, 27*(3), 370–375.

Snyder, L. H., et al. (1978). Wandering. *Gerontologist, 18,* 272–280.

Tappen, R. M. (1997). *Interventions for Alzheimer's disease: A caregiver's complete reference.* Baltimore, MD: Health Professions Press.

Thomas, D. R. (1988). Assessment and management of agitation in the elderly. *Geriatrics, 43*(6), 45–53.

Young, S. H., et al. (1988). Managing nocturnal wandering behavior. *Journal of Gerontological Nursing, 14*(5), 6–12.

Chapter 9

Falls and the Use of Mechanical Restraints

LEARNING OBJECTIVES

- To identify risk factors for resident falls
- To identify interventions to help prevent resident falls
- To identify the risks of using restraints with demented residents
- To list alternatives to the use of restraints as well as safe methods of employing them

---

PRETEST

Place a "T" before true statements, an "F" before false statements, and a question mark before those you don't know.

_____ 1. Restraints are the best method of protecting demented residents.

_____ 2. Only about 10% of nursing home residents fall each year.

_____ 3. A risky time for resident falls is right after admission to a nursing home.

_____ 4. Residents with lower extremity weakness are less likely to be injured when they fall.

_____ 5. Residents seldom fall in familiar places like their bedroom.

_____ 6. OBRA-87 forbids the use of any form of restraints in long-term-care facilities.

_____ 7. Residents often fall without hurting themselves.

_____ 8. The cost of caring for incontinence may go down when restraint use is reduced.

_____ 9. Assuring the bed is the right height so that the resident can easily get into it or out of it is a good way to reduce falls.

_____ 10. Demented residents may become more agitated when mechanically restrained.

Many of the most noteworthy changes in long-term care in recent years have been the result of the Nursing Home Reform Act found in the Omnibus Budget Reconciliation Act of 1987 (OBRA-87). This act states that residents in nursing homes have the right "to be free from physical or mental abuse, corporal punishment, involuntary seclusion, and any physical or chemical restraints imposed for purposes of discipline or convenience and not required to treat the resident's medical symptoms" (p. 165). On the basis of this mandate, a new set of regulations for restraint use in nursing homes was developed, effective October 1990 (Burton, German, Rovner, Brant, & Clark, 1992) As a result of these regulations, many long-term-care facilities have embarked on programs to reduce the use of mechanical and chemical restraints while, at the same time, striving to maintain the safety and well-being of their residents.

One of the primary reasons mechanical restraints have been used in long-term-care settings is to reduce the risk of falls among the frail elderly residents. The first part of this chapter looks at falls and what we know about their causes and the characteristics of those who fall. The second part of the chapter looks at mechanical restraints, alternatives to their use, and under what circumstances mechanical restraints may be "required to treat the resident's medical symptoms."

FALLS

Resident falling is one of the most significant safety issues facing a long-term-care institution. According to Tinetti (1997), more than

Answers: 1-F, 2-F, 3-T, 4-F, 5-F, 6-F, 7-T, 8-T, 9-T, 10-T.

50% of ambulatory nursing home residents fall each year. Although very few of these falls lead to significant physical injury (about 4% of falls among nursing home residents result in fractures, and 11% result in serious soft-tissue injuries) (Tinetti, 1997), a fall is still a traumatic event. Fear of falling can be as disabling as an actual physical injury to an older person. An initial fall may lead to what Hendrich, Nyhuis, Kippenbrock, and Soja (1995) refer to as the "fall event cascade" of decreased mobility, decreased activities of daily living, decreased body system functioning, and increased susceptibility to disease, which can lead to death. Tideiskaar (1993) refers to the "downward spiraling effects of falls" in which a fall leads to a loss of confidence and therefore restricted ambulation. This may lead to another fall—perhaps causing a broken hip, which leads to bed immobility and the complications associated with bed rest—which leads to death.

From the perspective of caregivers and the long-term-care facility, a fall presents a legal liability. A resident fall is one of the most common reasons physicians, nurses, and hospitals are sued for medical negligence (Hendrich et al., 1995).

WHO FALLS

Several characteristics have been found to be common to nursing home residents who are at high risk for falling (Ouslander, Osterweil, & Morley, 1997). These include such demographic characteristics as being a woman and being older than 75. Being newly admitted to a facility is also a risk factor. Having had a previous fall within a year puts a resident at a higher risk of having another fall. Moderate to severe dementia, perhaps because it leads to a reduced safety awareness, also puts a resident at greater risk for falling. Physical/medical problems contributing to an increased risk of falling include: gait instability and poor balance; multiple physical disabilities; poor vision; muscle weakness, particularly weakness in the lower extremities; having more than four medications prescribed; routine use of psychotropic drugs; postural hypotension; and urinary incontinence. Requiring assistance with basic activities of daily living (ADL) and being unable to perform more than two basic ADL tasks is also associated with an increased risk of falls.

Tinetti (1997) emphasizes that falls most often result from "the accumulated effects of multiple impairments and disease." Nursing home residents have, on average, a higher number of impairments than persons living in the community and thus are more likely to fall.

WHERE AND WHEN DO RESIDENTS FALL

Most falls of long-term-care residents occur in the bedroom, the bathroom, or the dining room (Cali & Kiel, 1995; Tideiksaar, 1993). The high number of falls occurring in these areas reflects the amount of time residents spend in them. The more time a person spends in a room, the more likely, if the person is to fall, he or she will fall in that room.

Falls occur at all times of the day and night. Many occur at night when a resident gets up out of bed to go to the bathroom. However, Cali and Kiel (1995) found that most falls that resulted in fractures occurred during the daytime and early evening hours. Since most falls occurred when residents are ambulating, and more residents are up and walking around during the daytime and evening, there is a higher likelihood of falls occurring during these times. Many falls also occur when residents are transferring from one position to another, for instance, from bed to wheelchair, on or off the toilet, from wheelchair to a regular chair. As many as 30% of falls occur when a resident is in the process of sitting down or standing up (Schnelle et al., 1994).

ENVIRONMENTAL FACTORS ASSOCIATED WITH FALLS

Most modern long-term-care facilities have been designed with fall prevention in mind. Many hazards have been removed, and environmental factors associated with falls in the community (stairs, icy sidewalks) are rarely encountered by long-term-care residents (Tinetti, 1997). However, there are still environmental factors, even within the long-term-care setting, that can contribute to resident falls. These include: shiny, slippery floors; wet floors (Cali & Kiel, 1995); chairs and beds that are too high, too low, or that roll; walking aids such as canes or walkers; and problem footware such as ill-fitting shoes and untied shoelaces.

Miss Kiernan lived in a long-term-care facility. She was slow moving and stiff from Parkinson's disease but she was able to walk and do most self-care tasks for herself. One day, she leaned from her bed to push shut the window. Someone had neglected to lock the wheels of her bed. As she pushed on the window, the bed rolled backward and Miss Kiernan fell to the floor. She broke her right arm near the shoulder and dislocated her left shoulder. She became completely helpless, and only after months of physical therapy and occupational therapy was she able to do any self-care tasks for herself.

FALL-RISK ASSESSMENT

One way of managing risk of falls among residents of a long-term-care facility is by assessing each resident for characteristics that would put them at a higher risk for falls. There are several assessment devices in the literature that were developed to be used to evaluate fall-risk status. Some of these scales use information that correlates with fall risk, which can be found in the case record. Some are fairly straightforward observational scales, asking the resident to perform a behavior sample in a standardized way and observing and rating the performance. Training and experience are required of the person administering the assessment in order to rate residents in a consistent manner. Some scales combine a case record review with a performance sample and may also draw information from a physical examination of the resident to develop an assessment of fall risk.

The following are brief descriptions of a few of the available scales to evaluate fall risk.

• Fall Risk Index—(Developed by Tinetti, Williams, & Mayewski, 1986), this scale combines information from a chart review, a physical examination, and a performance test called the Performance Oriented Mobility Index. The Performance Oriented Mobility Index evaluates both gait and balance with such tasks as rising from a chair, walking a short distance, and standing with eyes closed. Thapa, Gideon, Breckman, Fought, and Ray (1996), in evaluating several clinical and biomechanical measures as fall predictors, found the balance subscale of the Performance Oriented Mobility Index to be one of the best measures to independently predict future falls in residents that had already fallen once.

• Get Up And Go (Mahtias, Nayak, & Isaacs, 1986)—Besides having a catchy title, this is one of the simplest performance-based measures of mobility and balance (Andersen, Rothenberg, & Zimmer, 1997). It is comprised of getting up from a straight chair with armrests, walking about 10 feet, turning around, returning to the chair and sitting down. The resident's performance is rated by someone who is trained and experienced with the test.

• Fall Risk Checklist (Tideiksaar, 1993)—This scale includes information on risk factors found in the case record or through physical examination along with an evaluation of actual performance of transfer and ambulation tasks. Performance is observed in both the bedroom and the bathroom.

• Safety Assessment for the Frail Elderly (SAFE; Schnelle et al., 1994)—This scale is a performance assessment of transitioning and walking. It evaluates 10 components relevant to transitioning and 13 components relevant to walking. The items include evaluation of the resident's awareness of safety (e.g., locking the wheels of the wheelchair before transitioning) as well as observation of physical performance (e.g., evaluation of balance and movement ability).

• Hendrich Fall Risk Model (Hendrich et al., 1995)—This scale assigns "risk points" to various resident characteristics such as confusion/disorientation, altered elimination, and so on to get a Final Risk Score. The model also suggests interventions that are appropriate for different levels of Final Risk Scores. These suggested interventions include the use of soft restraints for the highest risk levels when lower level interventions have been unsuccessful.

• Physical Functioning and Structural Problems—Section G of the Minimum Data Set (MDS)—The MDS is required by the Health Care Finance Association (HCFA) to be completed for residents of nursing homes receiving Medicare and Medicaid. It is completed on newly admitted residents as well as at regular intervals subsequent to admission or when there is a change in health status. The MDS includes a section on physical functioning and structural problems, the responses to which could trigger the completion of a Resident Assessment Protocol (RAP) for falls (Ouslander et al., 1997). This evaluation, since it has already been done for the residents in many facilities, might be a good way to screen residents for level of fall risk.

STEPS TO MINIMIZE FALL RISK

Once you have done a fall-risk assessment and you know which residents are at greater risk of falling, there are several things you or your facility can do to minimize the risk of falling.

Environment

The environment of the long-term facility, particularly in the bathrooms and the bedrooms, should be looked at for potential hazards and for ways of enhancing safety features.

• Lighting—Lighting is very important. Sufficient light that is glare free with night lights for nighttime illumination is a requirement. There should be light switches by doorways so that residents do not have to walk through a darkened room to turn on a light. Natural lighting is preferable to artificial lighting during the daytime.
• Floors—Floor surfaces should be slip resistant and carpet edges securely tacked or taped down. Pathways between bed and bathroom, or bed and doorway, should be free of obstacles including low-lying objects that are difficult for residents to see and therefore easy to trip over.
• Furnishings—Attention should be paid to furnishings as well. Beds should be low in height, or adjustable to a low height, and stable to allow safe, independent transfers. Special consideration should be given to bed (side) rails. Many falls have occurred when residents tried to climb over bed rails to get out of bed at night. Full-length bed rails are especially problematic. If bed rails must be used, it is suggested that devices that are one-half to three-fourths the length of the bed be installed instead of full-length bed rails. This allows residents space to get up off the bed if they need to, but also keeps them from accidentally rolling out of bed in their sleep (Tidieksaar, 1993). Some residents use bed rails for support, to help turn themselves over, to pull themselves up, or to hold onto when they stand up. A one-half to three-quarter length bed rail serves well for this purpose.

Chairs should be untippable and equipped with armrests. Tables should be sturdy and able to support a person's balance when leaned on. Movable, over-the-bed tables on wheels should not be used. Shelving for possessions should be reachable by the resident without having to stand on tip-toe or on a chair.

• Safety devices—Safety devices such as hand rails and toilet and tub/shower grab bars should be securely fastened at appropriate heights. Elevated toilet seats are safer for resident transfers. Call bells should be easily reachable by residents who need assistance in transitioning.

Tideiksaar's book (1993) has extensive information on environmental safety enhancements for long-term-care facilities.

Resident Interventions

There are several approaches to interventions with residents that will help reduce their risk of falling.

• Instruction—Residents can be taught to move more safely and avoid falls. Even residents with dementia, with frequent reminders and supervision, can learn to move more safely. Instruction should include emphasizing the importance of wearing proper footwear with nonskid soles and with laces tied. Persons with postural hypotension should be instructed about getting up slowly to assure sufficient blood flow to the head. Residents can be taught and reminded to call for assistance, to avoid wet areas on the floor, to follow safety measures such as locking their wheelchairs before transferring, etc. Residents can be instructed in safer ways to fall (e.g., relaxing and rolling) and what to do if they should fall (stay where they are and call for help).

• Physical Conditioning—Another resident intervention to reduce fall risk is to improve the resident's strength and flexibility. Physical therapy programs can improve strength and mobility by having residents exercise, including using weights to strengthen legs and arms. Recently researchers have shown that even very frail elders can increase their strength and improve their gait through very intensive exercise programs. However, so far it is unclear if such exercise programs actually lead to a reduction in falls (Rubenstein & Wieland, 1993; Tinetti, 1997). Physical therapists can instruct residents in improving their gait so that they would be less likely to trip. They can also instruct residents in the proper use of ambulation assistive devices such as walkers, canes, or specially fitted shoes. A resident who is using such devices properly is less likely to fall or to cause others to fall.

• Medication Adjustment—An effort can be made to reduce the number of drugs a resident is taking, since an increased risk of falls is highly correlated with taking four or more medications. Staff should also make an effort to avoid the use of medications that have an increased likelihood of falls as a side effect.

Nursing Interventions

In addition to evaluating residents by doing fall-risk assessments, nursing care staff can perform other interventions to reduce the risk of falls in their facility.

• Increased awareness—Direct care staff can identify residents who are at increased risk of falling with some identifying device such as a pin or a wristband which distinguishes those who have been evaluated to be a high risk for falling. Staff can also place a sticker on a resident's chart and/or a sign of some sort on the door to the room of a resident who is a high fall risk. High risk residents can be moved to rooms nearer the nurses station so that they can be more closely observed.

• Intensification of Care—Direct care staff can pay special attention to newly admitted residents, helping them become accustomed to the facility. Staff can follow a program of taking residents to the bathroom on a more frequent and regular basis, as many falls occur when residents try to get themselves to the bathroom. Staff can carefully monitor residents for signs of acute illness (which can lead to an increased risk of falls) and provide closer supervision when a resident is ill. Residents should be re-evaluated for level of fall risk after an acute illness. Nursing staff can increase the safety of residents who climb out of bed by lowering the bed rails, by lowering the height of the bed and/or by padding the floor around the bed. Increasing the staff-to-resident ratio is another intervention that has been found to reduce fall risk.

• Inservices—Nursing care staff should have education in fall and injury prevention on a regular basis.

MECHANICAL RESTRAINTS

Mechanical or physical restraints are devices, material, and equipment that: (a) are attached to or are adjacent to the individual's body; (b) prevent free bodily movement to a position of choice (standing, walking, turning, sitting); and (c) cannot be controlled or easily removed by the individual (Stilwell, 1988; Tideiksaar, 1993). Mechanical restraints include sleeveless vests (tie vests) and sleeved jackets, waist belts and sheets, pelvic supports, wrist and ankle ties, mitts, geriatric chairs, and wheelchairs with fixed tray tables. Side rails, especially full-length ones, on beds are sometimes included as a mechanical restraint.

USE OF MECHANICAL RESTRAINTS

As recently as the late 1980s, mechanical restraints were commonly used in nursing homes for a variety of reasons. Resident safety was the most frequently cited reason (Magee et al., 1993) for the use of restraints. Restraints were often used with residents who wandered, who went into other residents' rooms, who were agitated and disruptive, or who interfered with medical treatments (by, for instance, pulling out urinary catheters, nasogastric tubes or IVs), who were at risk of falling. At times, restraints were used to control or discipline an unruly, agitated resident or to keep someone put in a safe place until staff could attend to his or her needs. Research showed that between 25% to 85% of residents of nursing homes were restrained (Evans & Strumpf, 1989; Tinetti, Liu, Marottoli, & Ginter, 1991). Many researchers (Evans & Strumpf, 1987; Post, Krasnausky, Grossman, & Lynch, 1994) found the use of mechanical restraints excessive. They found that being restrained led to increased agitation especially among residents with dementia. Residents who were restrained showed an increase in rate of cognitive decline over time when compared to residents who were not restrained (Burton, German, Rovner, & Brant, 1992).

Mr. Farrelli was a difficult resident. He had had a head injury in an automobile accident as a young man and had very poor impulse control. He was very unsteady on his feet, but would still try to get up and walk independently. Several times he had fallen without injury, and the staff at the long-term-care facility where he lived were very concerned that he would fall and break a hip. This was especially a concern at night when he would try to get up out of bed when there were fewer staff available to monitor him. To keep him safe, the staff decided to use mechanical restraints, in addition to the bed rails, to keep him in bed. They tried a soft belt but he was able to get out of it. They tried a tied jacket but somehow he was able to untie it and squeeze out of it. To prevent him from untying the restraint, they applied wrist restraints so that he could not use his hands to untie the jacket restraint. Because Mr. Farrelli was aggressive and would kick staff who came to give him care during the night, ankle restraints were ordered for the safety of staff. Thus, in the interest of safety, Mr. Farrelli spent each night restrained with a tie jacket, wrist restraints, ankle restraints, and bed rails. This continued until the facility started a program of restraint reduction and alternatives to restraint were sought to assure his and the staff's safety.

The use of restraints are themselves associated with injury and even death (Dube & Mithcell, 1986; Miles & Irvine, 1992).

Mrs. Anvers lived in an adult care home and was fairly independent. She became ill with pneumonia and had to be hospitalized for IV antibiotic therapy. To protect her from falling and to keep her in bed, she was restrained with a tie vest and the side rails were raised on her bed. When the nurse on rounds checked her, she was found hanging over the side rail, suspended by the tie vest. She was dead.

The use of restraints has been associated with such physical consequences as skin breakdown and bed sores, reduction in appetite, contractures, urinary and fecal incontinence, fecal impaction, nerve damage, circulatory problems, and edema (Brundgardt, 1994; Souren, Franssen, & Reisberg, 1995; Sundel, Garrett, & Horn, 1994; Tideiksaar, 1993).

In addition, the use of restraints is seen as dehumanizing and undignified to the residents under restraint. In their 1993 article, Kane, Williams, Williams, and Kane indicate that there has been a major shift in attitudes in what constitutes good care. This is a change from a paternalistic, "medical science knows best," and "physical safety is the most important issue" approach to one of person-centered care, individualized treatment approaches, and increased concern about the loss of dignity and potential psychological harm the use of restraints can impose. OBRA-87 came about as a result of this change in attitude.

RESTRAINT USE UNDER OBRA-87

The Nursing Home Reform Act of OBRA-87 does not forbid the use of mechanical restraints in nursing homes. It does set strict guidelines for their use. It forbids the use of restraints for the convenience of staff or to "punish" problematic behavior. However, in some cases, the use of mechanical restraints may be the only way to protect a resident from injuring himself or herself or others. For those circumstances the following guidelines are suggested (adapted from Post et al., 1994).

• Restraints should not be used routinely. There should be no standing orders for mechanical restraints to be used as needed. There must be a physician order specific for the situation requiring the restraint.

• The benefits and risks associated with restraint use must be explained to the resident or the family and their consent for use must be obtained.

• The least restrictive restraint that will handle the situation should be ordered by the physician for a specified time period. There must be frequent checks for the proper application and to assure the resident's comfort.

• Restraints are required to be released every two hours for resident exercise and toileting.

• In emergency situations, restraints may be applied without consent, but for a very limited time and under very specific conditions.

• Staff should be involved in ongoing education programs regarding the appropriate use of restraints, alternatives to restraint use including positive behavioral management techniques, and manipulations of the environment.

REDUCING THE USE OF MECHANICAL RESTRAINTS

Since the OBRA-87 regulations have gone into effect, many long-term-care facilities have embarked on efforts to reduce the use of mechanical restraints. To be successful these efforts have usually required a change in the system, a change in the philosophy and attitudes of administrators, direct care staff and family members. Burton, German, Rovner, Brant, and Clark (1992) found restraint use was more associated with attitudes of the staff than with characteristics of the resident such as dementia or mental illness. Kramer (1994) discusses the need for direct care staff to be "socialized" to resist the idea of restraint use rather than to think first of using restraints. These changes in philosophy and attitude are brought about not only by educational and in-service programs but also by actually implementing a restraint reduction program and seeing that it does work (Ejaz, Folmar, Kaufmann, Rose, & Goldman, 1994).

Implementing a successful restraint reduction program requires several components (Mahoney, 1995; Kramer, 1994; Janelli, Kanski, & Neary, 1994):

- Education—including information about the dangers of restraint use as well as alternatives to their use.
- Involvement of all levels of staff—administrators, physicians, direct care nursing staff, support staff. Everybody must be informed about the program, educated about the program, and understand their role in the changes being made.
- Multidisciplinary advisory team—to plan strategies for removing restraints and to develop alternatives for more difficult cases.
- A trial-and-error, one step at a time approach—removing restraints from the easiest cases first.
- Involving families—in educational programs as well as decisions about restraint use with their loved one.
- Environmental and staffing adjustments.

Some nursing homes have been able to reduce their use of mechanical restraints to below 5% (Cohen, Neufeld, Dunbar, Pflug, & Brewer, 1996; Ejaz et al., 1994). However, a nationwide study found that, in general, mechanical restraints were being used for 21% of nursing home residents (Cohen et al., 1996). Although this is certainly an improvement from pre-OBRA-87 days, it shows there is still room for further reductions.

A motivation for long-term-care facilities to continue to reduce the use of restraints is that research studies have shown there are benefits to restraint reduction in addition to the improved comfort and happiness of residents. Most restraint reduction programs have been done with little need for increased staffing and minimal extra cost (Cohen et al., 1996; Mahoney, 1995). There may be a savings in staff time that was previously used in checking and periodically releasing restraints as required and in doing ADL care for residents who could not do for themselves because of being tied down. One study (Mahoney, 1995) even noted a monetary savings when restraint use was reduced because of the significant reduction in the need for incontinence supplies.

ALTERNATIVES TO THE USE OF MECHANICAL RESTRAINTS

One of the reasons commonly given for the continued use of mechanical restraints was that there were no alternatives. However, when forced by OBRA-87 to seek alternatives to restraints, necessity and creativity came to the forefront and alternatives were developed. Some of these alternatives, it is true, turned out to be as restrictive of movement as the traditional restraint they were designed to replace (Schnelle & Smith, 1996). They meet the letter, but not the spirit of the law. A Geri-lounge chair in the lounge position is more restrictive to a resident's mobility than a wheelchair even when the resident uses a restraining seatbelt while in the wheelchair. Self-releasing fasteners such as Velcro fasteners on lap belts are not less restrictive if the demented resident is unable to learn how they work. On the other hand, exchanging a pelvic restraint in a wheelchair for a safety belt the resident can release may be truly liberating and a step toward independence. Thus, alternatives to mechanical restraints must be individualized; they must be looked at as to whether they enable the resident to be more independent or restrict the resident to the same or greater degree than the previous restraint (Cohen et al., 1996).

The following are some suggested alternative approaches to the use of mechanical restraints:

• Philosophy—The nursing home administration and direct care staff can adopt the attitude that residents have the right to individualized care, to be involved in decisions about their care, and to have the right to take some risks (Brungardt, 1994; Kane et al., 1993; Post et al., 1994; Radar & Donius, 1991).
• Environment—

♦ Alarms—Alarms can be used to help keep track of people who wander or to signal when residents, who are unable to walk safely, are trying to get up on their own. Examples include exit door alarms, bed and chair alarms, body position alarms.

♦ Furniture—Experimenting with different kinds of furniture has led to innovative ways of reducing restraints. Examples include: rocking chairs, beanbag chairs, Adirondack chairs, beds closer to the floor, and use of positioning devices like wedge pillows.

♦ Doors—Doors can be fitted with alarms or with latching mechanisms that are too difficult for demented residents to learn, or doors can be disguised by mirrors, plants or other objects set in front of them, or a cloth strip across the doorway fastened with Velcro.

♦ Safe walking areas such as a circular indoor path and an enclosed outdoor area.

• Restorative programs—Programs to restore strength and functioning in residents can often solve problems for which mechanical restraints were previously used. Examples include frequent toileting; walking and exercise programs; physical therapy for gait training, limb strengthening, and balance improvement; as well as diversional activities.

• Staffing—Staff can be deployed differently so that, for instance, there is more staff available for frequent toileting and to provide activities when the residents are most active.

SUMMARY

In this chapter we have discussed falls, a significant safety problem for elderly long-term-care residents, and what steps can be taken to reduce the risk of falls and serious injuries. We have also discussed the changes that have come about with the Nursing Home Reform Act of OBRA-87. The use of mechanical restraints, which previously were extensively used to prevent residents from falling, has been significantly limited by OBRA-87. We discuss the appropriate use of restraints and alternatives to their use.

LEARNING EXERCISES

1. Most of us fall occasionally. Think of the last time you fell. What factors caused the fall to happen, for example, environmental

conditions or obstacles, risk taking, footwear, etc.? List all the causative factors you can think of for your fall. Then list what factors could have been changed to prevent the fall. Have you made these safety changes? How can you apply your insight into your own behavior to improve your residents' safety?

2. Have someone place restraints on you while you are seated in a wheelchair. Sit there for an hour without saying anything. Discuss your feelings.

3. Think of a resident for whom physical restraints are currently being used. List the steps you would take to reduce the use of restraints with this resident.

POSTTEST

Place a "T" before true statements, an "F" before false statements, and a question mark before those you don't know.

_____ 1. Restraints can cause strangulation and bed sores.

_____ 2. About 50% of nursing home residents fall each year.

_____ 3. Certain medications can increase the resident's risk of falling.

_____ 4. A physician's order, specifying the restraint to be used and the length of time it is to be used, is required for using restraints.

_____ 5. Family members are never involved in decisions about whether or not to use mechanical restraints.

_____ 6. Reducing the use of mechanical restraints is too expensive to be practical in most nursing homes.

_____ 7. All levels of staff, from administrators to cleaners, need to be involved in a restraint reduction program.

_____ 8. Residents who fall suffer a serious injury, such as a broken hip, in about 50% of falls.

_____ 9. Caregivers change their attitude about the need for mechanical restraints when they see that reducing restraints actually works.

_____ 10. Dementia residents cannot benefit from exercise programs designed to increase strength and mobility.

Answers: 1-T, 2-T, 3-T, 4-T, 5-F, 6-F, 7-T, 8-F, 9-T, 10-F.

REFERENCES

Andresen, E., Rothenberg, B., & Zimmer, J. G. (Eds.). (1997). *Assessing the health status of older adults.* New York: Springer Publishing Co.

Brungardt, G. S. (1994). Patient restraints: New guidelines for a less restrictive approach. *Geriatrics, 49,* 43–50.

Burton, L. C., German, P. S., Rovner, B. W., & Brant, L. J. (1992). Physical restraint use and cognitive decline among nursing home residents. *Journal of the American Geriatrics Society, 40,* 811–816.

Burton, L. C., German, P. S., Rovner, B. W., Brant, L. J., & Clark, R. D. (1992). Mental illness and the use of restraints in nursing homes. *Gerontologist, 32,* 164–170.

Cali, C. M., & Kiel, D. P. (1995). An epidemiologic study of fall related fractures among institutionalized older people. *Journal of the American Geriatrics Society, 43,* 1336–1340.

Cohen, C., Neufeld, R., Dunbar, J., Pflug, L., & Brewer, B. (1996). Alternatives to physical restraints. *Journal of Gerontological Nursing, 22,* 23–29.

Dube, A. H., & Mitchell, E. K. (1986). Accidental strangulation from vest restraints. *Journal of the American Medical Association, 256,* 2725–2726.

Ejaz, F. K., Folmar, S. J., Kaufmann, M., Rose, M. S., & Goldman, B. (1994). Restraint reduction: Can it be achieved? *The Gerontologist, 34,* 694–699.

Evans, L. E., & Strumpf, N. E. (1987). Patterns of restraints: A cross-cultural view. *Gerontologist, 27,* 272A.

Evans, L. E., & Strumpf, N. E. (1989). Tying down the elderly: A review of the literature on physical restraints. *Journal of the American Geriatrics Society, 37,* 65–74.

Hendrich, A., Nyhuis, A., Kippenbrock, T., & Soja, M. (1995). Hospital falls: Development of a predictive model for clinical practice. *Applied Nursing Research, 3,* 129–139.

Janelli, L. M., Kanski, G. W., & Neary, M. A. (1994). Physical restraints: Has OBRA made a difference? *Journal of Gerontological Nursing, 20,* 17–21.

Kane, R. L., Williams, C. C., Williams, T. F., & Kane, R. A. (1993). Restraining restraints: Changes in a standard of care. *Annual Review of Public Health, 14,* 545–584.

Kramer, J. D. (1994). Reducing restraint use in a nursing home. *Clinical Nurse Specialist, 8,* 158–162.

Magee, R., Hyatt, E. C., Hardin, S. B., Stratmann, D., Vinson, M. H., & Owen, M. (1993). Use of restraints in extended care and nursing homes. *Journal of Gerontological Nursing, 19,* 31–39.

Mahoney, D. F. (1995). Analysis of restraint-free nursing homes. *Image, The Journal of Nursing Scholarship, 27* 155–160.

Mathias, S., Nayak, U. S. L., & Isaacs, B. (1986). Balance in elderly patients: The "Get-up-and-Go" test. *Archives of Physical Medicine Rehabilitation, 67,* 387–389.

Miies, S. H., & Irvine, P. (1992). Deaths caused by physical restraints. *Gerontologist, 32,* 762–766.

Omnibus Budget Reconciliation Act of 1987. (1987, December 22). Public Law 100-203.

Ouslander, J. G., Osterweil, D., & Morley, J. (1997). Gait disorders and falls. *Medical care in the nursing home* (2nd ed., pp. 251–273). New York: McGraw-Hill.

Post, D. C., Krasnausky, P., Grossman, H. D., & Lynch, D. (1994). The reduction of restraint use in the nursing home. In M. K. Aronson (Ed.), *Reshaping dementia care* (pp. 94–108). Thousand Oaks, CA: Sage.

Rader, J., & Donius, M. (1991, March/April). Leveling off restraints (Restraints in the 90's). *Geriatric Nursing,* pp. 71–73.

Rubenstein, L. Z., & Wieland, D. (Eds.). (1993). *Improving care in the nursing home.* Newbury Park, CA: Sage.

Schnelle, J. F., MacRae, P. G., Simmons, S. F., Uman, G., Ouslander, J. G., Rosenquist, L. L., & Chang, B. (1994). Safety assessment for the frail elderly: A comparison of restrained and unrestrained nursing home residents. *Journal of the American Geriatrics Society, 42,* 586–592.

Schnelle, J. F., & Smith, R. L. (1996). To use physical restraint or not? *Journal of the American Geriatrics Society, 44,* 727–728.

Souren, L. E. M., Franssen, E. H., & Reisberg, B. (1995). Contractures and loss of function in patients with Alzheimer's Disease. *Journal of the American Geriatrics Society, 43,* 650–655.

Stilwell, E. M. (1988). Use of physical restraints on older adults. *Journal of Gerontological Nursing, 14*(6), 42–43.

Sundel, M., Garrett, R. M., & Horn, R. D. (1994). Restraint reduction in a nursing home and its impact on employee attitudes. *Journal of the American Geriatrics Society, 42,* 381–387.

Tideiksaar, R. (1993). *Falls in older persons: Prevention and management in hospitals and nursing homes.* Boulder, CO: Tactilitics.

Thapa, P. B., Gideon, P., Breckman, K. G., Fought, R. L., & Ray, W. A. (1996). Clinical and biomechanical measures of balance as fall predictors in ambulatory nursing home residents. *Journal of Gerontology, Medical Sciences, 51A,* M239–M246.

Tinetti, M. E. (1997). Falls. In C. K. Cassel, H. J. Cohen, E. B. Larson, D. E. Meier, N. M. Resnick, L. Z. Rubenstein, & L. B. Sorenson (Eds.), *Geriatric medicine* (3rd ed., pp. 787–799). New York: Springer-Verlag.

Tinetti, M. E., Liu, W. L., Marottoli, R. A., & Ginter, S. F. (1991). Mechanical restraint use among residents of skilled nursing facilities: Prevalence, practice and predictors. *Journal of the American Medical Association, 265,* 468–471.

Tinetti, M. E., Williams, T. F., & Mayewski, R. (1986). Fall risk index for elderly patients based on number of chronic disabilities. *American Journal of Medicine, 80,* 429–434.

SPECIAL ISSUES

Chapter 10

Caring for the Younger Resident

LEARNING OBJECTIVES

- To know the types of conditions and illnesses that may cause younger individuals to become nursing home residents
- To learn how dementia is often a part of the conditions that lead younger persons to become nursing home residents
- To understand why younger residents can often present special problems to staff in nursing homes
- To identify effective approaches in caring for the younger resident
- To learn ways to cope with the stress of caring for the younger resident

PRETEST

Place a "T" before true statements, an "F" before false statements, and a question mark before those you don't know.

_____ 1. Only younger people can get AIDS.
_____ 2. Persons with multiple sclerosis may have memory problems.
_____ 3. AIDS dementia may be accompanied by a slowing or clumsiness in movement.

___ 4. Younger residents are more like nursing home staff and so are easier to care for.

___ 5. A person with memory problems can be helped by having calendars and clocks easily available.

___ 6. Very few of the younger residents in a nursing home have conditions that include dementia as a symptom.

___ 7. The human immunodeficiency virus (HIV) appears to directly attack brain cells.

___ 8. Younger residents in nursing homes haven't experienced as many losses as older residents.

___ 9. It's easy to keep your perspective when caring for a younger resident and not get emotionally involved.

___ 10. Household bleach is very effective in disinfecting items and areas contaminated by human immunodeficiency virus.

WHO ARE THE YOUNGER NURSING HOME RESIDENTS?

Most residents of nursing homes are very old. However, there are usually a few young residents in any large nursing home. In fact, younger residents may become more common in long-term care as many facilities are including rehabilitation units or children's units in the range of services they offer. At times these younger residents can present special problems to the long-term-care staff.

Younger people enter nursing homes for the same reasons older people do: they have a seriously debilitating physical condition or disease that requires nursing care, and they lack sufficient social supports to be maintained in the community. Some nonelderly adults' need for long-term care could have resulted from accidents with severe spinal cord or brain injury, heart attacks and strokes, multiple sclerosis, cerebral palsy, developmental disabilities, and chronic mental illness (Dhooper, 1997). Often some element of dementia is present in these younger individuals as part of their condition. Children requiring long-term care are most often those with developmental disabilities (Dhooper, 1997).

Answers: 1-F, 2-T, 3-T, 4-F, 5-T, 6-F, 7-T, 8-F, 9-F, 10-T.

CHARACTERISTICS OF DEMENTIA IN THE YOUNGER RESIDENT

Although dementing illnesses are much more prevalent in late life, the types of conditions that require a younger person to seek long-term care often have a dementia component. Head injuries, stroke, and other neurological conditions that affect younger people as well as the elderly have a good chance of causing symptoms of dementia. Whether or not dementia is present and how it is demonstrated is dependent on what area of the brain is affected. Debilitating diseases also, such as multiple sclerosis (MS) or Huntington's disease, usually have dementia symptoms such as memory problems (Marsh, 1980; van den Burg et al., 1987). Learning new material is more difficult for individuals with MS than retrieving stored material. Therefore, MS residents might not be able to learn their way around a new environment but can easily recall details of their past. The severity of cognitive symptoms increases in the more advanced stages of MS (Marsh, 1980; van den Burg et al., 1987). Because MS residents in nursing homes are likely to be at a quite advanced stage of the disease, they may need frequent reminders and memory aids such as clocks, calendars, and an orientation board.

The relative lack of sensory and social stimulation that is part of illness and of life in an institution can lead to a sensory deprivation that can cause dementia-like symptoms. As with an older person, a younger person who is ill, dependent on others for care, and away from home may react with depression. The individual may appear slowed down, lethargic, and disoriented, as if the person were demented. Depression may actually be the source of these symptoms.

How best can the caregiver approach the younger resident? One answer is to treat this resident in the same way any resident is treated—as a needy human being who requires caregiving services. However, this is a caregiving situation that is complicated by unusual feelings and behaviors. Caregivers must remain aware that individuals with dementia also have major role changes with relocation to a nursing home; these role changes can often be difficult because of changes associated with the relocation itself (e.g., new environments, caregivers, schedules) as well as the changes associated with ongoing declines secondary to dementia (Kelley, Swanson, Maas, & Tripp-Reimer,

1999). We will explore some of the issues that often seem to make care of younger residents in a long-term-care facility so difficult.

RESIDENTS' FEELINGS

The losses an older person may experience when entering a long-term-care facility are often highlighted. We understand the older person's need to mourn the loss of a home, independence, and family members. A younger person also experiences these losses. In addition, a younger person may have additional "losses" or missed opportunities to deal with. The younger person may be mourning the chance of ever having a normal life with a career, family, love, and success. The younger person may just have started on these life tasks when accident or illness struck. The need to readjust life goals, view of self, and perception of the future may cause very strong negative feelings. Although the initial readjustment may be difficult, the resident's ability to cope with a severe disability improves over time (Hirschwald, 1997).

> *Sam Johnston was a man in his early 30s when he was admitted to a VA Nursing Home Care Unit. He had been working as a computer programmer, although for the past few years, this work was part time as his MS progressed. By the time Sam was admitted, his fiancee had left him, he was on disability, and he could no longer even feed himself. Sam had a bright smile for everyone, though staff could tell he was hiding a very deep hurt.*

Younger residents may feel resentment at having to live among sick older people, who don't share their lifestyle, desires, or interests. The music, movies, and recreational interests of younger persons are very different from those of older adults, for whom most nursing home programs are geared. A younger person may really resent being in a setting where so much of the leisure activity is designed for another age group.

A younger resident may be dealing more acutely with issues of sexuality and sexual needs than older residents. Although older people have sexual feelings, sexual drives are stronger in the young. It is important to maintain a professional relationship and give clear messages to avoid potential problems in this area.

Although many older people feel ready to face death after living a full life, a younger person with a terminal illness may be angry and resentful of this turn of fate. Finally, younger residents may be dealing with feelings of isolation and ostracism. They may even feel shame for having contracted a disease that forces them to be dependent on others and live in an institution outside the mainstream of society.

STAFF MEMBERS' FEELINGS

Although we may accept that younger residents have stronger or different feelings than older residents, it may be harder to accept that staff react or feel differently toward younger residents. However, a good caregiver does adjust the style of care to the needs of each resident. Therefore, it is natural that one would treat a younger resident differently than an older resident. It is also natural that one might experience different feelings toward a younger resident.

"Countertransference" is a psychoanalytic term that can apply to a caregiving situation. It means that the caregiver, usually unconsciously, thinks of the resident as if the person were really another individual important in the caregiver's life. The caregiver thinks of the resident as having the personality and reactions of this other person and responds to the resident as if the resident were this person. This can occur with the older resident when caregivers see the resident as a parent or grandparent. However, the young resident is more near the age of the caregiver. So the caregiver may think of the resident as if the resident were a brother or sister, child, or even spouse. By unconsciously thinking of the resident as if the resident were someone important in the caregiver's life, the caregiver may attribute feelings and motivations to the resident that are true of the "significant other," but not necessarily true of the resident. For example, when a young male resident does not comply with a caregiver's request, it reminds the caregiver of caring for a younger brother who willfully disobeyed and got the caregiver into trouble with his or her mother. The caregiver's reaction to the resident's noncompliance may consequently be much stronger and more upsetting than if the caregiver were truly objective about the resident.

Another element in the caregiver's reactions to younger residents is identification—thinking of the resident as the same as oneself. When a resident is near the caregiver's age, the caregiver can't help but feel, "There but for the grace of God go I." This can be a scary feeling. It can also make the caregiver feel very sorry for the resident. The caregiver may make a special effort to provide out-of-the-ordinary services to the resident. The caregiver might even try to turn the resident into a personal friend. If the resident doesn't reciprocate, or demands more special favors, or begins to ignore the rules, the caregiver may feel hurt or betrayed and blame the resident. This is the risk of ignoring the need for professional distance between staff and residents.

> Joan was a woman in her 40s who had suffered a spinal cord injury in an auto accident and was quadriplegic. She had a young daughter and had been divorced by her husband after the accident. She lived in a skilled nursing home with occasional visits to her sister's home where her daughter lived. Several staff members on the unit befriended her. After all, she was just like them except for her disability. When they went on break, they would include Joan and take her with them to the staff break room for a cigarette. They would talk among themselves as friends. In this way Joan began to feel that she was not "just a resident," and she also learned personal details of the staffs' lives. When Joan repeated these personal stories to others, the staff members were shocked that she would do such a thing. When she expected and demanded to be taken to the staff break room for a cigarette, they were amazed at her nerve and boldness. When the staff suddenly put strict limits on Joan's behavior and privileges, Joan felt hurt and betrayed. There were upset and unhappy feelings on both sides.

This could have been prevented by recognizing from the beginning the need to maintain a professional type of relationship with residents. Caregivers can be warm, friendly, and even affectionate with residents and still maintain a distance that protects against unrealizable expectations and false hopes. To maintain such a distance, caregivers would want to refrain from disclosing details of their personal lives. Caregivers would also want to provide comfort to the resident, rather than have the resident provide emotional support to the caregiver. It would also be important to avoid overreacting to tragedies in the resident's personal life, and to prevent oneself from "getting in the middle" of resident-family problems. The caregiver must also be fair with time, giving each resident in their care, young and old, the time necessary to meet the resident's needs.

RESIDENTS' FEARS

Another issue that makes an impact in the care of the younger resident is fear. The resident has fears that must be acknowledged. Probably fear of the illness, dependency, and what the future holds are the greatest fears that younger residents will have. Individuals respond to feelings of fear by withdrawing from others or by becoming uncooperative and irritable. A resident might even become aggressive as a result of fear—identifying everyone as the enemy and being suspicious of the motives of the caregiver. By understanding that fear is causing the resident to act in this way, caregivers can help calm and reassure the resident with emotional support. The individual will need to be reassured that he or she—with the exception of the disability—is the same person as before and will be treated in the same way to the extent possible (Hirschwald, 1997).

CAREGIVERS' FEARS

The caregiver may also experience fear in caring for residents. A younger resident, even when sick, may be physically more powerful than most older residents. If that younger resident is uncooperative or aggressive, the caregiver could realistically experience some fear of being hurt while caring for the person. For example, a study by Jacobs (1988) on caregiver burden, found that caregivers of people with traumatic brain injury report that behavioral, emotional, and cognitive problems are the most difficult to handle (as cited in Smith & Schwirian, 1998). A caregiver could also experience the fear of identification—if this could happen to the younger resident, it could happen to me, now, not 40 years from now as with the older residents. This fear that "it could happen to me" may lead a caregiver to unconsciously avoid the younger resident and be more curt when providing care, so as to not get close to the resident and be reminded of this possibility.

RESIDENTS WITH AIDS

A group of younger individuals who may become increasingly numerous in long-term-care facilities are persons suffering from acquired immune deficiency syndrome (AIDS) (*Morbidity and Mortality Weekly Report,* 1998). One of the effects of infection by human immunodeficiency virus (HIV) is dementia. As this virus infects more persons and more of those infected begin to have symptoms of the disease, nursing homes are faced with large numbers of younger residents in need of nursing care and support.

The disease syndrome resulting from HIV infection has become a major public health problem, not only in the United States but also throughout the world. HIV attacks the immune system, destroying the body's ability to defend itself against infections and cancers it would normally conquer with ease. The virus is spread by direct contact with the blood or certain body fluids of infected individuals. Thus, the disease can be spread through intimate sexual contact, through infected, blood-stained needles, blood transfusions, and other sources of contact with the blood of infected individuals. The virus dies quickly when exposed to air. Household chlorine-based bleach is an effective disinfectant in its control (Durham & Cohen, 1987).

The growth and impact of the HIV/AIDS epidemic has taken an enormous toll—socially, emotionally and financially—at the individual resident level as well as the societal level. Although the trend of this disease in the United States has been to affect mainly people in a few high-risk groups (e.g., homosexual and bisexual men, intravenous drug users, and the sexual partners of infected individuals)—it has spread well beyond that realm. The disease has spread among heterosexuals, both male and female, young and old, White and non-White, drug users, and urban as well as rural areas (Dhooper, 1997). In fact, more than three out of four new HIV infections are a result of heterosexual transmission (Deren et al., 1997). Also, babies born to infected mothers are at high risk to contract the disease. The reported cases of AIDS actually understate the true extent of the epidemic because the time lag between infection with HIV and the development of AIDS can be quite lengthy (U.S. Department of Health and Human Services, 1995). Before the virus was discovered and its mode of transmission was known, infected individuals donated blood. Persons who had received infected blood or blood products developed AIDS. Some of those who contracted the disease through blood transfusions are elderly (Sabin, 1987; Weiber, Mungas, & Pomerantz, 1988). Recent advances in the treatment of HIV have slowed or reversed the progress of the disease for many of those infected. Thus, the advent of improved antiviral drug regimens has moved us toward the goal of dealing with HIV as a manageable chronic disease (Morrison, 1999), similar to diabetes, which must constantly be treated with a variety of medications.

   As the number of affected individuals increases and their need for skilled nursing care remains high, it seems likely that nursing homes will continue to be used for the care of people with AIDS. Services that long-term-care facilities provide to residents with AIDS may include palliative care—as in hospice, short-term recuperative stays posthospitalization until the resident is able to return home, and for treatment of people who are no longer safe living alone (Klein, Botticello, & Kramer, 1996). Therefore, service providers in hospital, outpatient programs, and long-term-care facilities will continue as a part of the treatment and care of the victims of AIDS and similar other diseases (Dhooper, 1997). The AIDS dementia complex is just one of the many aspects of this infection that will require care.

AIDS Dementia Complex

Persons infected with HIV have been found to have several possible causes for a dementia syndrome. In some cases the dementia is secondary to an opportunistic infection (i.e., an infectious agent that has taken the opportunity of the HIV depressed immune system to infect the body). Infectious agents that frequently affect the brain and cause cognitive or emotional symptoms include toxoplasmosis, cytomegalovirus, herpes encephalitis, and disseminated tuberculosis (Howe, 1996; Navia & Price, 1987; Ostrow, Grant, & Atkinson, 1988). Cancers in the brain can also cause dementia symptoms. In addition, many HIV-infected individuals experience depression, which can result in cognitive symptoms. But it has also been found that the HIV itself can directly attack brain cells, causing damage that leads to symptoms of dementia (Howe, 1996; Navia, Jordan, & Price, 1986); AIDS dementia complex has been observed to occur in 60% to 80% of AIDS patients (Dhooper, 1997). Early in the course of the disease, the symptoms include difficulty concentrating, impaired recent memory, slowing of thinking, slowing and clumsiness of movement, slurring of speech and deterioration of handwriting, and impaired motor function (Stine, 1996). Many times these symptoms are assumed to have been caused by depression (Buckingham & Van Gorp, 1988; Stine, 1996). However, in the case of AIDS dementia complex, these symptoms can progress to a severe global dementia, inability to speak, paraplegia, and incontinence (Navia et al., 1986). Researchers have found that the damage from HIV is primarily located in the white matter and subcortical structures of the brain with relatively little involvement of the gray matter or cortex. In addition, it appears that treatment with azidathymidine (AZT) and protease inhibitors can reverse the damage to the brain as shown in magnetic resonance imaging (MRI) studies (Howe, 1996; Melton, Kirkwood, & Ghaemi, 1997; Ostrow et al., 1988). Treatment can improve the quality of life of AIDS dementia sufferers and extend the time of relative well-being and mental functioning for the two-thirds or more of AIDS patients who experience a dementia in addition to their other problems.

When caring for a resident with an infectious disease such as HIV, caregivers may experience a very stressful fear of contracting this disease as a result of normal duties. Because the disease is not completely understood and some people are skeptical of the reassurances of scientists and health officials, many caregivers will fear caring for persons with a disease such as HIV. This fear can be overcome by education and provisions made by the health care facility for using appropriate infection control procedures. Educational programs have been developed and books have been written especially for health care workers caring for AIDS patients (Durham & Cohen, 1987). Much research has been done monitoring health care workers and family members continually exposed to HIV infected individuals (deVita, Hellman, & Rosenberg, 1997). People do not become infected with HIV through casual contact with infected individuals. The greatest risks to health care workers are from accidental needle sticks with contaminated needles. These include disposable syringes, IV line/needle assemblies, prefilled cartridge injection syringes, winged steel needle IV sets, vacuum tube phlebotomy assemblies, and IV catheters (Stine, 1996). Prolonged, unprotected contact with blood and blood-contaminated body fluids (Durham & Cohen, 1987) will also transmit the virus. Immediate treatment with HIV medications has been found to help prevent HIV infection in cases of accidental needle sticks and other unprotected exposures to the virus.

The treatment regimens of residents with HIV/AIDS are becoming very complex, and it takes experience and a great deal of knowledge to provide the adequate level of care for these patients (Morrison, 1998). With continuing-education requirements for license renewal, caregivers are becoming more informed about modes of virus transmission, infection control procedures, and treatment options for those infected. Staff are also gaining experience in providing care to AIDS residents. Thus, fear of caring for residents with AIDS is lessening.

THE ART OF CARING FOR THE YOUNGER RESIDENT

Providing good care is an art. It involves being skillful and confident and being sensitive to the special needs of each individual resident. Caring for younger residents requires perhaps even more sensitivity and awareness of the resident's special needs and the caregiver's own reactions.

It is important to keep in mind the special feelings and fears that younger residents may have. If feelings of sadness and anger seem to overwhelm the person, caregivers should inform other staff (e.g., a social worker, charge nurse, chaplain, or physician) who might be able to provide counseling or other treatment that would help. Try to find activities and entertainment that would be of interest to the younger resident and more "age appropriate." Although it is important to be friendly, warm, and accepting of the younger resident, it is equally important to maintain an appropriate professional distance. This makes it easier in the long run for both the caregiver and the resident.

The younger resident may experience feelings of shame, guilt, and abandonment. These feelings are caused both by their condition as well as the living situation. It is up to the caregiver to recognize these feelings and help the resident change them by showing respect and empathy. Also, residents with an infectious illness such as HIV need to feel accepted rather than ignored or shunned. Infection control procedures should be explained to the resident and carried out in a courteous, matter-of-fact manner. Actually, infection-control practices also help protect the resident. Because of a poorly functioning immune system, many residents are very susceptible to other infections.

The resident may be having memory and other brain problems as a result of the disease. The person may not recall directions that have been given or incidents that have happened. Like an older person, a younger resident may need calendars and clocks to remain oriented. The younger resident may show poor judgment in certain situations. This does not necessarily indicate a willful lapse in appropriate behavior and should be considered part of the dementia. However, depression is also expressed with a slowing down, forgetfulness, and lack of interest in things. Depression should be considered as an explanation for unusual behavior. Such symptoms should be brought to the attention of the physician for appropriate treatment.

SUMMARY

There are usually a few young residents in a nursing home. It often appears that they are more difficult to care for than the more typical older resident. They have special characteristics and problems that affect the outlook of the caregiver. This may lead to difficulties in the resident/caregiver relationship. However, if the caregiver is aware of these special needs and problems and is sensitive to personal reactions, the caregiver can approach the younger resident in a confident, supportive, professional manner and provide excellent care.

LEARNING EXERCISES

1. Imagine yourself, right now, with some illness or physical condition that requires care in a long-term-care facility. What aspects of your present life would be most important for you to maintain while you were a resident of the facility? Consider leisure activities, music, or television shows you like, family relationships, sexual intimacy, religious observances, and so on. How could these needs be met if you were a resident in a long-term-care facility? How would you cope if these needs could not be met?
2. Discuss your understanding of infection-control procedures, and how these would apply to caring for an AIDS resident. Investigate where you could get more information about AIDS. Discuss what kind of staff training and educational programs a facility should provide when AIDS patients become residents of the facility.
3. Discuss people's feelings about using infection-control procedures (masks, gloves, etc.) during resident care. Role-play how you would approach a resident with whom you were using infection control measures. Explain to the "resident" why you are using the procedures. Then discuss how it felt to make this

explanation. Receive feedback from the class as to what was effective and ineffective about the way you presented the topic.

4. If you are a caregiver, think of and share with the class experiences you may have had in caring for a resident who was considerably younger than the majority of residents at your facility. What were the pleasures and rewards in caring for this resident? What were the most difficult aspects of the care? Can you identify any countertransference or identification issues that may have been factors in your care of this individual? Would you change anything in the way you approach the younger resident?

POSTTEST

Place a "T" before true statements, an "F" before false statements, and a question mark before those you don't know.

_____ 1. Education is the best way to help caregivers get over their fear of caring for AIDS residents.

_____ 2. The severity of the memory loss often seen in multiple sclerosis has no relationship to the progression of the disease.

_____ 3. Young residents in nursing homes can fit in easily because they are too sick to miss the things most people their age are doing.

_____ 4. Recognizing the different feelings a younger resident may cause in a caregiver can help the caregiver cope with them better.

_____ 5. More than half the people with AIDS have cognitive impairment at some time in the course of their illness.

_____ 6. If you think of the resident as if the person were yourself, you are identifying with the resident.

_____ 7. A professional attitude in caregiving necessarily interferes with a warm, friendly approach.

_____ 8. A resident who takes advantage of a caregiver's friendly approach may be misinterpreting the caregiver's intentions.

_____ 9. Participation in bingo and music from the 1930s may turn off younger residents.

____ 10. Even a resident with AIDS needs to have reasons for infection precautions explained.

REFERENCES

Buckingham, S. L., & Van Gorp, W. G. (1988). Essential knowledge about AIDS dementia. *Social Work, 33,* 112–115.

Deren, S., Kotranski, L., Beardsley, M., Collier, K., Tortu, S., Semaan, S., Lauby, J., & Hamid, R. (1997). Crack users in East Harlem, New York, and Philadelphia, Pennsylvania: HIV-related risk behaviors and predictors of serostatus. *American Journal of Drug and Alcohol Abuse, 23,* 555–567.

deVita, V. T., Hellman, S., & Rosenberg, S. A. (1997). *AIDS: Biology, diagnosis, treatment, and prevention* (4th ed.). New York: Lippincott-Raven.

Dhooper, S. S. (1997). *Social work in health care in the 21st century.* Thousand Oaks, CA: Sage.

Durham, J. D., & Cohen, F. L. (Eds.). (1987). *The person with AIDS: Nursing perspectives.* New York: Springer Publishing Co.

Hirschwald, J. F. (1997). Rehabilitation of a quadriplegic adolescent: Regional spinal cord injury center. In T. S. Kerson & Associates (Eds.), *Social work in health settings: Practice in context* (2nd ed., pp. 353–374). Binghamton, NY: Haworth Press.

Howe, M. (1996, July 26). Opportunistic infections (Part XXVIII). Neurological complications. *AIDS Information Newsletter.*

Joyce, C. (1988). Assault on the brain. *Psychology Today, 22*(3), 38–44.

Kelley, L. S., Swanson, E., Maas, M. L., & Tripp-Reimer, T. (1999). Family visitation on special care units. *Journal of Gerontological Nursing, 25*(2), 14–21.

Klein, W. C., Botticello, P. J. Jr., & Kramer, J. (1996). People with AIDS as residents: Preparedness and acceptance by Connecticut long-term-care facilities. *Journal of Health & Social Policy, 8*(2), 25–40.

Marsh, G. G. (1980). Disability and intellectual function in Multiple Sclerosis patients. *Journal of Nervous and Mental Diseases, 168,* 758–762.

Melton, S. T., Kirkwood, C. K., & Ghaemi, S. N. (1997). Pharmacotherapy of HIV dementia. *Annals of Pharmacotherapy, 31,* 457–473.

Morbidity and Mortality Weekly Report. (1998). Diagnosis and reporting of HIV and AIDS in states with integrated HIV and AIDS surveillance—United States, January 1994–June 1997. *47,* 309–314.

Answers: 1-T, 2-F, 3-F, 4-T, 5-T, 6-T, 7-F, 8-T, 9-T, 10-T.

Morrison, C. (1998). HIV/AIDS units: Is there still a need? *Journal of the Association of Nurses in AIDS CARE, 9*(6), 16–18.

Navia, B. A., Jordan, B. D., & Price, R. W. (1986). The AIDS dementia complex: I. Clinical features. *Annals of Neurology, 19,* 517–524.

Navia, B. A., & Price, R. W. (1987). The acquired immunodeficiency syndrome dementia complex as the presenting or sole manifestation of the human immunodeficiency virus infection. *Archives of Neurology, 44,* 65–69.

Ostrow, D., Grant, I., & Atkinson, H. (1988). Assessment and management of the AIDS patient with neuropsychiatric disturbances. *Journal of Clinical Psychiatry, 49,* 14–22.

Sabin, T. D. (1987). AIDS: The new "great imitator." *Journal of the American Geriatrics Society, 35,* 467–468.

Smith, A. M., & Schwirian, P. M. (1998). The relationship between caregiver burden and TBI survivors' cognition and functional ability after discharge. *Rehabilitation Nursing, 23,* 252–257.

Stine, G. J. (1996). *AIDS update 1996.* Upper Saddle River, NJ: Prentice Hall.

U.S. Department of Health and Human Services. (1995). *Hospital resource use by HIV-infected females: Provider studies research note 25* (AHCPR Publication No. 96-N001). Rockville, MD: Public Health Service, Agency for Health Care Policy and Research.

van den Burg, W., et al. (1987). Cognitive impairment in patients with Multiple Sclerosis and mild physical disability. *Archives of Neurology, 44,* 494–501.

Weiber, P. G., Mungas, D., & Pomerantz, S. (1988). AIDS as a cause of dementia in the elderly. *Journal of the American Geriatrics Society, 36,* 139–141.

Chapter 11

Working with Families of Dementia Residents

LEARNING OBJECTIVES

- To describe the stresses of family caregiving
- To outline five stages that caregivers go through when providing care to the dementia resident at home
- To acknowledge the family caregiver's need to protect the self-esteem of the dementia resident
- To understand that family caregivers often continue their feeling of responsibility even after their family member is placed in a nursing home
- To help the family deal appropriately with guilt
- To suggest ideas that family members can use to improve their nursing home visits
- To realize the importance of frequently orienting both resident and family to each other
- To identify alarming situations for families and strategies for dealing with them
- To realize the importance of a staff/family partnership

PRETEST

Place a "T" before true statements, an "F" before false statements, and a question mark before those you don't know.

____ 1. Most families will place their demented relatives in a nursing home.

____ 2. When families place their demented relative in a nursing home, they mainly feel relief.

____ 3. Most family caregivers feel they are very good at caring for the demented individual.

____ 4. Taking care of a person with AD at home usually lasts for no longer than one year.

____ 5. Families are often embarrassed by the behavior of their relative with dementia.

____ 6. Families feel it is important to maintain the self-esteem of their demented relative.

____ 7. Middle-aged women sometimes feel like a sandwich, caught between caregiving responsibilities from top to bottom.

____ 8. Over time, family caregivers can get physically sick themselves from their caregiving responsibilities.

____ 9. Guilt can cause a family member to never visit their demented relative.

____ 10. Family visits are best if they involve lots of talk and conversation with the resident.

CASE STUDIES

Mr. and Mrs. Johnson take care of their 3-year-old grandson while his mother works. Two other grandchildren, aged 10 and 12, come over after school for several hours. Mr. Johnson knows that his 70-year-old wife is very forgetful and demanding. Increasingly, he has to help her with simple everyday tasks like bathing and choosing what to wear. He also has to watch her carefully, because she will forget that the stove or iron is turned on. Because he is diabetic and has problems with walking, he has asked his grandchildren to help take care of Grandma. They have given up afterschool activities and time with friends to help out. They sometimes have to help with grooming and feeding tasks. They fear that some day they too will become a child again like their grandmother. The older boy has nightmares about it. The children's mother is quite upset about the situation, but can't afford other childcare arrangements. Besides, her mother needs the help. However, her son's coach, aware of the

_____

Answers: 1-F, 2-F, 3-T, 4-F, 5-T, 6-T, 7-T, 8-T, 9-T, 10-F.

*boy's problems, has pressed for other health care arrangements for the grand-
mother. The family soon decides to place Mrs. Johnson in a nursing home.*

*Mrs. Bennett, after raising four children, worked hard to get a masters degree
in education at the age of 47. She became a guidance counselor in high school,
greatly enjoying her job. However, after 5 years, Mrs. Bennett's husband,
aged 60, showed symptoms of dementia. Within 6 months, he needed a full-
time caregiver. Mrs. Bennett, after much soul searching, gave up the job she
loved to take care of her husband. She has been proudly giving him 100% of
his care, with little help from children or other relatives for 3 years. Increasingly,
her husband has become a problem. He is violent, will not eat regularly, and
recognizes nobody, not even his wife. He paces constantly and sleeps fitfully,
usually only during the day. Recently, he became incontinent. Mrs. Bennett,
after much discussion with her family doctor, who was concerned about her
stress and depression, finally agreed to place her husband in a nursing home.
However, her children have been arguing with her about this decision.*

These are some of the heartaches and crises that caregiving families
experience every day. Although the staff person in a long-term-care
facility may sometimes feel that families are dumping their problems
onto the nursing home, families have instead stretched themselves to
the limit, usually for far too long. In fact, two-thirds of families with
a dementia resident don't institutionalize their family member (Rabins,
1988). Those who do usually feel significant guilt and concern. Family
caregivers often believe that no one can care for their relative as well
as they can (Zarit & Zarit, 1986). Because of this belief, they have
often refused help for years from community resources or from other
family members or friends. They believe that their elderly relative
won't accept anyone else for assistance with caregiving. Minority families often prefer to keep family members home as long as possible, so
they can offer special foods, folk remedies, conversation in the native
language, involvement in religious festivities, or because of cultural
beliefs about illness (Espino & Lewis, 1998).

STAGES OF FAMILY CAREGIVING

Care for a demented person can last from a few to even 20 years.
During that period of time, the family caregiver has been under terrific
stress. Pollack (1988) describes the stages of caregiving experienced
by the family. In the initial stage of their loved one's disease, families

may experience denial—a sense of "This isn't happening; the doctors must be wrong." Ross and colleagues (1997) found that about 20% of families do not recognize that their loved one is demented. They can also, before the diagnosis is made, feel frustration with the person. A wife might say to herself, "Why doesn't he try harder?" and she might show impatience and anger.

In early and even later stages of the disease, the person can have "good" days when memory is improved. This causes the family to feel a kind of false hope, as there is no hope of improvement in many kinds of dementias. After such a false hope, the family's hopes can be dashed. It is important for family to appreciate the good days but realize that progressive deterioration is going to happen. What causes good days? We don't know, but it may be that the patient is more rested and so has more energy to function somewhat better.

As the person's disease progresses, the family member may feel increasing embarrassment about the person's behavior. The individual with AD loses inhibitions, and so may become very sexual, may refuse to take a bath, may dress in strange ways, and may even become violent. This can cause the family to move to the second stage, that of isolation. Friends and acquaintances may feel uncomfortable when visiting, and so may cut down on their visits. Family members may feel they really can't invite anyone to the house because their loved one is acting so strangely. And they can't get out of the house to get some respite because they can't leave the elderly person alone, and no one else can really cover for them. Few people are qualified to act as "adult sitters," and even if they were, families are reluctant to use them. Although there may be many relatives in a family, usually only one is the major caregiver. Other family members may be denying there is a problem or may feel guilty about not helping out more, so they tend to keep away. The elderly person with AD may forget who these family members are, and so may feel anxious around them, causing, in turn, anxiety and feelings of incompetence in people who might want to help. And so the primary caregiver is stranded at home. Rarely getting out or having any kind of fun, the caregiver begins to feel worn out. The caregiver may feel like a martyr. Some people enjoy the martyr role, but others may not be able to cope.

One important function of the caregiver at this stage is to protect the Alzheimer patient's self-esteem (Bowers, 1988). The caregiver tries to say and do things in such a way that AD individuals not realize they are being helped or guarded. This is a very important responsibility for the caregiver. Family members often resent hospital or nursing home staff who baby their loved one. They do not always like hearing their loved one called "Honey" or "Gramps." They are not comfortable with the idea that their loved ones are forced into activities that they do not wish to participate in. It calls attention to the negative changes in the elderly person.

The adult child who is the caregiver may have additional problems. Her spouse and children may feel neglected by her. She may feel like a "sandwich," having caregiving responsibilities for both the older and younger generations. She may have fights with her brothers and sisters, feeling that they should be sharing more of the load. Long-buried conflicts (Mom loved you more than me, so why am I the one who has to do this?) may resurface. Often, the middle-aged or older caregiver has to give up a job to provide full-time care. This can cause financial hardship for the family.

The next caregiving stage is stage three: resentment. At this point, the caregiver is providing almost total care for the patient. This can be very physically draining. Aronson (1988) found that family caregivers have increased blood pressure, heart attacks, and depression. Caregivers may be feeling lonely, exhausted, angry, and restless. Their loved one may never give them a moment of peace or privacy. One family caregiver complains, "He follows me around all the time. If I even go to the next room, he gets anxious. I never even get the chance to go to the bathroom in privacy." The family caregiver can resent this change in lifestyle and feel tremendous depression. The caregiver can also be saying to herself, "Why me? What did I do to deserve this?"

One sad aspect of providing all this care is that seldom do Alzheimer patients even appreciate it. They may have lost the capacity to show affection and gratitude. They may, by this time, have lost the ability to talk clearly, so that the family caregiver has lost a companion. A very shocking thing to caregivers occurs when the Alzheimer patient does not recognize the caregiver, even after all that has been done for them. The patient may even accuse the caregiver of being an intruder in the house. The caregiver may also feel guilty about feeling resentment, thinking perhaps that the caregiver owes this amount of care to a loved one.

The next stage is that of letting go. By this time, the family caregiver is feeling so burdened that an alternative is needed to full-time caregiving. Depending on community resources, some caregivers use adult day care services. However, transportation can be a problem. Others have someone come regularly into the home to help, although at times the demented person may not fully accept this caregiver. The family member too may feel that this help is not as good as what she/he can provide. Others in the family may not be supportive of the primary caregiver's decision. There can be many conflicts among family members. A doctor or social worker can help the family make the best decision for all concerned.

In the last stage, the caregiver has made the decision to place the individual in a nursing home or made other caregiving arrangements. The caregiver feels both relief and despair—relief that at last all responsibility for care does not fall on the caregiver's shoulders, but despair that the caregiver's reason for living, the main purpose in life, is no longer there. She may feel overwhelming guilt for giving up on perceived responsibilities, yet secretly relieved about the chance for new experiences. The caregiver is mourning the loss of a loved one or the person who is no longer inside the body of the loved one. If the person with AD is placed in a nursing home, the caregiver usually maintains the feeling of responsibility. The caregiver continues to believe that no one can provide the kind and level of care that has been provided. The caregiver may feel worried that the loved one is not receiving adequate care. Sometimes, the caregiver spends a large amount of time at the nursing home, observing the kind of care the family member is receiving. Guilt about giving up the caregiving task may lead to a very critical attitude toward the nursing home staff. Or the caregiver may feel inadequate, realizing that the staff are actually providing better care than the caregiver did, and that the elderly person with AD is behaving better in the nursing home than at home. Zarit and Zarit (1986) suggest that placement shifts the burden but doesn't replace it.

Caregivers who place family members in nursing homes may replace the physically draining aspects of care with increased worries and emotions. Too, the caregiver may resent the loss of control over the resident. The family caregiver is no longer the one to decide what the resident eats, when the resident bathes, and so on. The caregiver has given up this decision-making power to the institution, and this may be frightening. The family caregiver may understand the loved one's likes and dislikes far better than the institution and may feel, rightly so, that no one is listening to suggestions and explanations.

The decision to place a loved family member in a nursing home is never easy. The "last straws" for family caregivers, causing them to make the placement decision, may include the person's wandering away, lack of sleep, violent or dangerous acts, or incontinence (Powell & Courtice, 1983). Unfortunately, nursing homes still have a very negative reputation with both older adults and their families. Very often, family members have promised their loved one that they will "never put them in a nursing home." Violating this promise can be very stressful. The financial costs can also be frightening. The nursing home may cost $50,000 a year or more. Other difficulties the family faces include the burden of visiting if the home is not close. The ethical decisions that must be made when the dementia resident gets physically sick also provide anxiety and guilt.

DEALING WITH GUILT

Guilt is a horribly unpleasant emotion. In order not to feel it, people will often behave in extreme ways. Some people will become a martyr, doing everything they can for the dementia resident. The family with a resident in the nursing home who takes this approach to dealing with guilt will visit all the time, even if this creates a hardship for themselves. Family will feel the need to take care of the resident and will be upset when others are doing what they feel deep in their hearts they should be doing. So nothing anybody else does is good enough. People who become martyrs will complain bitterly about the staff person's care of their family member. Staff members can't seem to do anything right. Not only will family members complain to them, family members will also complain to supervisors and to the administrator of the facility. It is very difficult for staff members to know that they are functioning to the best of their ability, and yet to be told that this is not enough, or is wrong or harmful to the resident. Knowing the reason for the constant criticism can help staff members be more understanding of the family. The best way to handle complaints is to listen carefully to them. A family member needs to feel understood. Staff members can also try to identify for the family members their feelings about the situation. One might say, "I know it must be really hard for you to care so much for your husband and yet not be able to do the things you used to do for him."

The other extreme approach that people use to deal with guilt is to avoid what is causing them this unpleasant feeling. Some family members will never visit the dementia resident, because if they visit, they feel guilt. They seem to go by the philosophy, "out of sight, out of mind." They deliberately try not to think about the resident. This way of coping also causes problems for the staff member, because the resident may be feeling very lonely and depressed. The resident may constantly say to you, "I want to go home. I want to go home. Where is my wife? Where are my children?" These questions are difficult to answer. They will probably make staff members feel uncomfortable. If the family member does come to visit, it is important for the visit to be as pleasant as possible. This can help cut down on a family's negative emotions, and they might visit more.

HELPING THE RESIDENT ADJUST TO ADMISSION

Rather than simply dropping off the person to be admitted at a strange facility, the family can ease this adjustment by bringing the person in for several visits before actually placing the person in the facility. The family can introduce the person to several staff on the unit the person will be placed on, allowing some familiarity with these new caregivers.

Although families worry that residents will have a difficult time adjusting, some residents adjust beautifully. They think the nursing home is a hotel or church or country club (Powell & Courtice, 1983). Other residents may take a very long time adjusting and be withdrawn or agitated for quite a while.

The family should bring in familiar objects and pictures that the resident can relate to to decorate the room. This can help the resident have a link with the past. The family will also feel more comfortable visiting if the resident's room seems familiar to them as well. The nursing home is not only strange to the new resident; it is also a strange place to family members. They must get used to long corridors, unfamiliar faces, disabilities and disfigurements in other residents, different odors. In a sense, they must also adjust to an institutional environment.

DEFINING THE PURPOSE OF VISITS WITH RESIDENTS

The family needs to have a purpose when they come to visit their relative, especially if verbal communication is difficult. If they come to discuss events or personalities, they may feel frustrated by the language problems of their loved one. The family could instead bring in photographs of the past to reminisce over with the resident. They could bring special foods to share. Staff members might encourage the family to take the resident on an outing, or to attend together a nursing home event. Often nursing homes will organize meals or parties that families are encouraged to attend. Other enjoyable activities include giving the resident a manicure, which encourages a lot of touching, or bringing in the grandchildren or pet for a visit. Of course, going for a walk is nice, or listening to music together and singing favorite songs. If the family is religious, it is meaningful to attend the chapel or services together, or to simply read aloud from the Bible. It is important to stress that family visits should be active and enjoyable. As the burden of providing heavy physical care is lifted, families may have more energy and willingness for meeting the emotional and social needs of the Alzheimer patient (Bowers, 1988). They may find that the relationship is improved and more meaningful than in the past.

When dementia residents lose their ability to interact with words, they can still understand nonverbal communication—touch, facial expression, voice tone (Hoffman et al., 1985). The family visitor should hug and touch the resident during the visit, talk with the person in a pleasant voice tone, and smile. Even though the resident may not understand the words, the positive message of love behind the words will be understood. This can greatly comfort the resident.

Of course, it is difficult for a family member who is feeling anxious and guilty to show these kinds of positive emotions. Staff members may need to calm the visitors before they see the resident. Visitors should be told how important it is for them to relax and feel better. Otherwise, they can make the resident feel agitated and uncomfortable. Often family visitors will comment, "What do I say to my loved one? She can't understand me at all." Tell the family that it is okay to say nothing. Simply being there with the resident, holding a hand, saying the person's name in a soothing way, perhaps singing a favorite song, all can make the person feel loved and needed.

Staff members should explain to the family that they should not overwhelm the resident with too many visitors at any one time. This can cause stress for the individual. One or two visitors at a time are plenty. Of course, there are special occasions when many family members will want to visit, such as a birthday or when grandchildren are home from college. Frequent, unhurried, but not overly long visits are pleasant for the resident. Just dashing in and out can disturb the resident, not allowing enough time to get used to the visitor.

Visiting can be an economic burden on the family if they rely on public transportation or live out of town. They may arrive at a facility feeling stressed because of a long commute or guilty that they can't visit more often because of transportation problems. Staff should express appreciation for the effort involved in visiting the facility.

ORIENTING PATIENT AND FAMILY

Away from the normal home setting, the resident may not recognize the family. This can make a family member feel very uncomfortable. The staff person needs to orient the resident on visiting day, reminding the resident over and over that the family is coming to visit, and reminding the resident of their names and roles. One might say, "Your husband, John Smith, is coming to visit you today," or "Your daughter, Mary Jones, will be visiting about 2:00 today."

The family also needs an update on the resident's condition. One might say, "Your mother has had an up and down week, but today she seems better." Orienting the family to the resident's condition helps prepare them for changes, either good or bad.

Staff may need to help the family feel comfortable doing less than they are used to for the resident. All of a sudden, former primary caregivers may have more free time than they know what to do with. They may want to spend every minute of their day at the nursing home. This can cause as much stress and fatigue as the former caregiving role at home. However, if this gives meaning and purpose to the former caregiver's life, staff must accept the person's need to continue giving to the resident.

Sometimes it is helpful for family members to get to know other residents in the facility, especially residents who have no family. They may enjoy chatting with these residents, feeding them, or running small errands for them. When their own family member doesn't recognize them or is having a bad day, the visitor can find comfort by talking with other residents in the nursing home.

Sometimes the family will be jealous of the new relationships that the resident makes in the facility, with other residents or staff. However, this is a sign that the resident is adjusting, and over time, the family realizes this.

PRESERVING SELF-ESTEEM

Bowers (1988) found that family members believe it is very important to preserve their loved one's self-esteem inside a nursing home. They believe this will do much to prevent depression. There are four kinds of caregiving that should be done to accomplish this. The first, maintaining family connectedness, is the responsibility of the family only. They accomplish this through frequent visits, reliving old times, celebrating birthdays, and so on.

The next three tasks for preserving self-esteem should be shared by family and staff. These include maintaining their relative's dignity, maintaining hopes, and giving some control over the environment to the resident. Families often believe that staff is not very good at these three tasks. If their loved one has a messy personal appearance, they can become quite upset at this loss of dignity. Also, when, for instance, physical therapy is cut off, the family believes this gives a sign to the resident of no hope for recovery. They feel very betrayed by a facility that takes their loved one out of rehabilitation-type activities. Families also resent when staff does not let the resident make choices about the timing of events. Sometimes staff also make residents feel that caring for them is a burden.

Families feel that it is their responsibility to educate the staff about the uniqueness of their relative—their likes, dislikes, accomplishments, disabilities. They feel it is important for staff to take these things into consideration when providing technical kinds of care. When families cannot be present, they use the resident's mood as an indicator of the kind of care staff is giving. If the resident is depressed, family feel that staff is giving poor care or has a bad attitude toward their family member. Families usually try to tell staff that something they have done must have caused this depression in their loved one. However, families sometimes feel that such complaining might make the staff angry. Staff should let the family know that open communication is appreciated.

FAMILY SUPPORT GROUP

Sometimes the facility will offer a family support group. Such groups are usually run by a social worker, psychologist, or nurse. In the group, family members are encouraged to voice their concerns and explain their frustrations, as well as share their positive emotions. Group members can comfort each other during bad times and offer suggestions as to how to deal with troublesome situations.

The Alzheimer's Association has chapters in most cities. Family members can join this group at any time. The Alzheimer's Association has speakers, supports research into the causes and cure for dementia, and offers group support. Staff of a nursing home will find many excellent ideas about how to manage their residents at these meetings. Staff often need support as much as families. The Alzheimer's Association can offer this kind of support. In some settings, the Alzheimer's Association staff will conduct support group meetings at the long-term-care facility. Usually the facility will join as a corporate member of the Association. Corporate members may also be eligible to send staff to free or low-cost training.

The National Institute on Aging and The National Institute of Nursing Research are sponsoring a major research program to develop new ways for family caregivers to deal with caregiving stress. The program is entitled REACH—Resources for Enhancing Alzheimer's Caregiver Health (Progress Report on Alzheimer's Disease, 1998). Families can be encouraged to use the program's Internet Web site to discover better strategies to manage their loved one with AD.

ALARMING SITUATIONS FOR FAMILIES

Families will usually be quite concerned if there is an incident or accident involving their loved one. Having their family member become physically hurt, usually as a result of a fall, is very upsetting. Often, they have placed their loved one in a facility to protect them from injury. If the resident is then injured in the new setting, the family can feel a lot of guilt, believing they have made a very poor decision about placement. Residents often fall in the first few weeks after placement. They are disoriented, confused, and have difficulty finding their way around. It is very important for staff members to spend a great deal of time in orienting the resident to the new surroundings. Staff must explain over and over again where to find things. Residents with Alzheimer's disease can learn over time to find important locations, but they need to be physically walked to these areas many, many times (McEvoy & Patterson, 1986).

It is also very worrisome for the family when their loved one wanders away from the facility. Families believe that the facility should be able to protect the resident from harm. They have placed their family member in a nursing home for protection and feel guilt if this cannot be successfully accomplished there. What is the point, they wonder, of all the trauma of nursing home placement if the nursing home can't take care of their loved one any better than they could at home?

It is upsetting for family members to be called and told about their loved one's strange behavior, such as getting into someone else's bed. Dementia residents will wander into other residents' rooms and touch their possessions very innocently. They are not doing it on purpose. They are simply lost or trying to find familiar landmarks. Families will feel better if they are asked for their advice as to how to manage some of the resident's more difficult symptoms, rather than merely complaining to the family about their loved one's more common behaviors such as wandering into other residents' rooms.

Families will sometimes feel very upset when their loved ones are placed on a special Alzheimer's unit. They may believe that the person is really not that impaired. Other families may feel excited, thinking their relative will improve on this unit. Then if no change occurs, they may feel very bitter.

Sometimes families have placed a family member in a nursing home for a physical condition. If the resident develops dementia in the facility, the family may blame the institution. A resident may develop a short-term delirium or acute confusion as a result of an illness. Relocation trauma or loss of familiar cues can also cause a dementia resident's confusion to worsen. At times, the side effects of medications can cause a dementia, as will a feeling of depression. However, some nondemented elderly residents will become demented over time as a result of their increased risk for developing illness with increased age. Once the resident is carefully assessed by a doctor and other conditions are ruled out, the family needs to be reassured that the nursing home placement is not the cause of the dementia. About 20% of the elderly persons over the age of 80 are at risk for developing dementia (Mortimer, 1983).

A PARTNERSHIP BETWEEN FAMILY AND STAFF

Bowers (1988) suggests that caregiving should be a "collaborative partnership" between family and nursing home staff. The Family Involvement in Care protocol is a well-developed program to clearly spell out family and staff roles (Maas et al., 1994). Family and staff should work together to provide high-quality care, which preserves the self-esteem of the resident. High-quality care means personalized care, taking into account the unique and special needs of the individual resident. Families love to be consulted about just what these special needs are, including the likes and dislikes of a resident, the strategies they used to manage certain behaviors, and for stories about their relative's past successes and accomplishments.

Edelson and Lyons (1985) suggest that nursing homes need families to provide another set of eyes and ears, watching for small signs that signal the beginning of an illness. They need families to provide ample clothes and shoes for residents, to help take residents to outside appointments and outings, to feed the residents who cannot eat on their own, or tempt their appetite with favorite foods. They especially need families to explain to them certain religious or ethnic practices that can influence a resident's behavior or preferences. But most important is the family's role in helping the resident feel loved and wanted despite changes in memory or personality.

By involving families rather than resenting them, staff members will have a much more enjoyable experience in providing excellent resident care. The appreciation received from a relieved family is one of the nicest aspects of a caregiver's job. Recently, an Italian wife of a resident brought into our unit one of the biggest batches of Christmas cookies we had ever seen. The cookies, including special Italian treats, lasted for several days, but her appreciation for our efforts will last a lifetime.

SUMMARY

Families of dementia residents are profoundly affected by their relative's disease. Usually a family member has cared for the person with dementia for many years. When it becomes necessary for the dementia resident to enter a long-term-care facility, the family caregiver must deal with many painful issues. These issues include the guilt of "abandoning" the person and of giving up full responsibility for the elder's care. Families should be enlisted as partners in the care of their institutionalized relative. They play an active role by helping preserve the identity of the demented person and by maintaining the person's well-being through attention, affection, and shared activities. Staff in long-term-care facilities should encourage and support families in their efforts to maintain ties with their loved one. By working together, staff and family can find the care of the resident easier and more enjoyable.

LEARNING EXERCISES

1. If you are a staff person, pair up with another staff person in your facility. One of you will take the role of an angry family member, upset about her relative's poor care. The other should practice listening carefully to the complaints, and identify the underlying emotions to the complainer. Switch roles.
2. Have you ever visited one of your own relatives in a hospital or nursing home? Did you notice any care that was inadequate? How did it make you feel? What did you do about it?
3. List as many ways you can think of that a nursing home can *lower* a resident's self-esteem. Discuss. How can family help the nursing home raise a resident's self-esteem?
4. Role-play a family member visiting a relative in a facility. Use the suggestions offered in this chapter to make the visit a quality visit.

POSTTEST

Place a "T" before true statements, an "F" before false statements, and a question mark before those you don't know.

___ 1. Family caregivers, over time, can feel tremendous resentment about their caregiving responsibilities.

___ 2. In early stages of AD, families sometimes refuse to accept the diagnosis.

___ 3. The primary family caregiver usually enjoys providing full-time care.

___ 4. The caregiver may be upset at the loss of control over the person with AD when the person is placed in a nursing home.

___ 5. Staff should try to ignore families when they are complaining about their relative's care.

___ 6. Families should participate in activities during their visits—going on a walk, singing songs, attending events with the resident.

___ 7. It is important to orient the family to the current condition of the resident.

___ 8. Maintaining the dignity of the resident is a shared responsibility of family and staff.

___ 9. If a nursing home resident falls or wanders away, families will often feel guilt about their decision to place the person in a nursing home.

___ 10. The Alzheimer's Association can be a support group for families and staff.

REFERENCES

Aronson, M. K. (1988). Patients and families: Impact and long-term management implications. In M. K. Aronson (Ed.), *Understanding and coping with Alzheimer's disease* (pp. 74–88). New York: Charles Scribner's Sons.

Bowers, B. J. (1988). Family perceptions of care in a nursing home. *Gerontologist, 28,* 361–368.

Edeslon, J. S., & Lyons, W. H. (1985). *Institutional care of the mentally impaired elderly.* New York: Van Nostrand Reinhold.

Espino, D. V., & Lewis, R. (1998). Dementia in older minority populations: Issues of prevalence, diagnosis, and treatment. *American Journal of Psychiatry, 6*(2), S19–S23.

Answers: 1-T, 2-T, 3-F, 4-T, 5-F, 6-T, 7-T, 8-T, 9-T, 10-T.

Hoffman, S. B., et al. (1985). When language fails: Nonverbal communication abilities of the demented. In J. T. Hutton & A. D. Kenney (Eds.), *Senile dementia of the Alzheimer type* (pp. 49–64). New York: Alan R. Liss.

Maas, M., Buckwalter, K. C., Swanson, E., Specht, J., Tripp-Reimber, T., & Hardy, M. (1994). The caring partnership: Staff and families of persons institutionalized with Alzheimer's disease. *American Journal of Alzheimer's Care and Related Disorders and Research, 9*(6), 21–30.

McEvoy, C., & Patterson, R. (1986). Behavioral treatment of the deficit skills in dementia patients. *Gerontologist, 26,* 475–478.

Mortimer, J. A. (1983). Alzheimer's disease and senile dementia: Prevalence and incidence. In B. Reisberg (Ed.), *Alzheimer's disease: The standard reference* (pp. 141–148). New York: Free Press.

Pollack, R. (1988). Dealing with the emotional turmoil of Alzheimer's disease. In M. K. Aronson (Ed.), *Understanding Alzheimer disease* (pp. 163–172). New York: Charles Scribners Sons.

Powell, L. S., & Courtice, L. (1983). *Alzheimer's disease: A guide for families.* Reading, MA: Addison-Wesley.

Progress Report on Alzheimer's Disease. (1998). Silver Spring, MD: ADEAR Center, National Institute on Aging.

Rabins, P. V. (1988). Psychosocial aspects of dementia. *Journal of Clinical Psychiatry, 49*(5), 29–31.

Ross, G., Abbott, R. D., Petrovitch, H., Masaki, K. H., Murdaugh, C., Trockman, C., Curb, J. D., & White, L. R. (1997). Frequency and characteristics of silent dementia among elderly Japanese-American men: The Honolulo-Asia aging study. *Journal of the American Medical Association, 277,* 800–805.

Zarit, S. H., & Zarit, J. M. (1986). Dementia and the family: A stress management approach. *Clinical Psychologist, 39,* 103–105.

Chapter 12

Special Care Units

LEARNING OBJECTIVES

- To define special care units (SCUs)
- To list the advantages and benefits of SCUs
- To identify the top 10 challenges of SCUs
- To suggest ways to enhance the physical environment of SCUs
- To suggest programming ideas for residents
- To list training needs of staff of SCUs

PRETEST

Place a "T" before true statements, an "F" before false statements, and a question mark before those you don't know.

_____ 1. A Special Care Unit (SCU) provides care to the chronically mentally ill.

_____ 2. SCUs improve resident ADLs.

_____ 3. SCUs should have an outside wandering area.

_____ 4. Staff on SCUs need special training in behavior management.

_____ 5. Long-term-care facilities use special care programs as marketing tools.

221

____ 6. SCUs are heavily regulated.
____ 7. Because residents are demented, there is little need for activity programs.
____ 8. Locked SCUs can feel like a prison to a demented resident.
____ 9. SCUs usually have good admission criteria.
____ 10. SCUs usually have adequate funding.

DESCRIPTION OF SPECIAL CARE UNITS

Special care units for demented persons are a recent development in the long-term-care industry. They have proliferated in nursing homes and assisted living facilities. Maas et al. (1998) suggest several reasons for this growth in SCUs: more individuals diagnosed with dementia, the difficult behavior management problems of demented individuals, consumer demand, and facilities wanting to attract private-pay residents. Such units usually house cognitively impaired residents who have a range of behavior problems. These units often have a system to prevent residents from wandering away. Only a handful of states have legislation regulating SCUs, but lobbying efforts of the Alzheimer's Association are encouraging more states to pass such legislation (Gerdner & Buckwalter, 1996). There are both advantages and disadvantages in placing dementia residents on such units.

ADVANTAGES OF SPECIAL CARE UNITS

Although special care units do not slow the deterioration of functional abilities or weight loss in residents (Phillips et al., 1997), their main benefits may be enhanced psychosocial well-being for residents and better staff morale. Also, many families prefer having their loved one placed on a "special" unit, and are willing to pay more to have them located on the SCU.

Well-designed and well-run special care units can be very satisfying to both residents and staff. On a good unit, staff choose to work there. There are an adequate number of staff. They are very well trained. There is an activities director designated for the unit. Activities are

Answers: 1-F, 2-F, 3-T, 4-T, 5-T, 6-F, 7-F, 8-T, 9-F, 10-F.

provided throughout the day, evening, and night, and are appropriate for cognitively impaired individuals. The design and furnishings have been carefully thought out. Residents have easy access to safe, pleasant, outdoor wandering areas. Food is well prepared and of an appropriate consistency, and there are enough staff to feed the residents without rushing. Snacks are available whenever residents are hungry. Administration supports the special care program, and families enjoy visiting.

Good special care units are rare, and they face a number of challenges.

CHALLENGES OF SPECIAL CARE UNITS

Hoffman and Kaplan (1998) list the 10 most common problems of special care units. These were identified by 77 participants at international conferences concerning dementia-specific care units.

- inadequate staffing
- lack of staff training
- inadequate programming for residents
- environment/design problems
- lack of support from other facility staff
- inadequate funding for dementia program
- lack of support from facility administration
- high staff turnover
- problems with families
- inadequate admission criteria

Inadequate Staffing

Administration must support a special care unit with adequate staffing. Using an adequate number of certified nursing assistants (CNAs) is particularly important. According to Maas and colleagues (1998), SCU residents need most assistance with eating and toileting, followed by watching out for their safety and socialization. The Office of Technology Assessment (1987) recommends one staff person to no more than six residents. The evening and night shift may also be a time of wakefulness on a dementia unit; these shifts need adequate staffing so that activities may be offered. CNAs should be trained in activity and simple rehabilitation programs so they can expand on and reinforce the work of the activities and rehabilitation staff.

Staff should be dedicated to the unit, as floating staff are often unaware of the special needs of dementia residents. Staff should be routinely assigned to the same resident. Certain staff are able to control and facilitate cooperation with particular residents.

Mr. Smith would eat for no one but a special LPN; she frequently had to come down during lunch from another unit to get Mr. Smith to eat.

Inadequate Training

Training must be offered continuously to all staff on the special care unit, and, in fact, to staff throughout a long-term-care facility. The trainer can be either the unit director, the nurse manager, a psychologist, or any other staff member competent to offer training. The trainer should both present information and model good skills with residents on the unit. All professions must be trained, including receptionists, secretaries, accountants, food service workers, and all other categories of staff. Staff need to be trained on every shift, and the trainer should monitor staff behavior on the floor to make sure that new skills are practiced during direct patient care.

The chapters of this book may serve as units for each session of training. Key topics to be addressed during training include:

- Overview of dementia
- Common sensory and memory problems
- Communication strategies
- Problem-solving and behavior management techniques
- Simple activities that dementia residents enjoy
- How to involve families

Each session should take about 30 to 45 minutes. Staff should practice their new skills both during the training session and also with residents after the session is completed. Stevens et al. (1998) suggest a self-monitoring checklist of new skills should be completed daily, to remind staff to use their new skills. This checklist should be turned in to the supervisor, and supervisors should reward staff for using their new skills.

Inadequate Programming

Locked units with little or no programming are essentially prisons. Programs are the most important feature of a special care unit. Activities keep the residents happily occupied and contribute to their sense of self-esteem and physical and mental health. Cohen-Mansfield, Marx, and Werner (1992) studied the activity involvement of dementia residents. In a 3-month observational study, they found that residents were involved in no activities at all 63% of the time and in structured activities very little of the time. They also noted that residents experienced more agitation when they were bored.

Activities directors should design programs that are appropriate for the cognitive level of the residents. Groups should be small and held in a quiet, enclosed area if possible. Quiet rooms or small day rooms without competing activities may be used. Activities may be held outside if weather permits. The following are examples of appropriate programs:

- activities of daily living—grooming or walking
- instrumental activities of daily living—folding towels, sweeping floors, setting tables, dusting and polishing furniture
- musical events—sing-a-longs, dances, making music with hand-held instruments, listening to favorite music
- sensory stimulation activities—cooking and baking, making popcorn, smelling flowers, touching objects of various textures, looking at pictures or family albums
- arts and crafts with nontoxic materials—coloring, water colors
- sports activities—balloon volleyball, ball toss, parachutes
- gardening
- spending time with facility pet
- community outings
- exercise to music
- relaxation group
- reminiscence group
- reading newspaper (when possible)

- playing favorite TV games, e.g., "The Price is Right"
- bingo
- sewing scraps of material
- a box full of things to tinker with
- hair brushing
- hand massage with lotion

Activities may be individualized to the special needs of residents. An accountant may enjoy a desk area with calculator, spreadsheets, stationery, and envelopes. A mother of many children may enjoy cuddling a baby doll. Buettner (1998) lists a variety of therapeutic recreational interventions for specific behavior problems. For example, depressed residents may benefit from spiritual activities, reminiscence, pet therapy, or exercise.

Poor Design

The most common concern regarding special care units is that of physical design. Many special care units are developed in spaces not originally intended for dementia programs. They may be on upper floors of a facility, which limits access to outdoor wandering areas. There may be safety concerns because of resident access to stairwells or busy streets. Long corridors, crowded spaces, inconvenient bathrooms, and busy nurses stations all contribute to resident disorientation and confusion. Poorly designed furniture, patterned wallpaper or carpets, high-glare floors, loud overhead paging, and easily accessible exits are also problems. Although some of these design defects may be addressed through renovations and retrofitting, some are not able to be fixed. Staff must work around these flaws.

Special care units should be homelike. Furnishings and interior design should be traditional, to remind residents of their homes from long ago. Dark wood, gold carpets, chintz fabric are reminiscent of home. Adequate lighting is essential. And natural lighting, from windows and skylights, is desirable. Loud noise should be kept to a minimum—TVs should not be left on; public address (PA) systems and loud alarms should not be used.

Inadequate Admission Criteria

Admission criteria that are clearly stated and followed are essential to a unit's success. Some units feel the pressure of maintaining a high census and so may admit inappropriate residents. This causes hard feelings among the staff. Other units do not have clearly defined criteria. Kaplan (1996) suggests the following admission criteria:

- a confirmed diagnosis of dementia
- a stable medical condition
- capability of participating in unit activities
- "absence of behavior disorders that are beyond the program's care or safety capacity"

This last criterion is particularly important. Residents with psychiatric problems may be very aggressive and violent. They may pose a safety risk to frail, elderly, dementia residents. Persons with criminal backgrounds may also be unsuitable for special care units.

Special care units are at risk for being sued unless their admission and discharge criteria are carefully followed.

Discharge criteria are also important. When residents become too physically frail to benefit from the program, the unit may decide to discharge them to a regular skilled nursing floor. However, some special care units have two levels of care—one for less impaired residents and one for total-care residents. The total care level needs less group activities, but should provide bedside programs.

Residents who become too aggressive to be managed on the unit, acting as a threat to themselves or others, may need to be discharged to a geropsychiatry unit in a hospital or other facility.

SUMMARY

Special care units should be "special." They should have well-trained staff, offer a safe, comfortable environment for residents, and have ongoing programs appropriate for persons with cognitive impairment. Inadequate staffing and staff training, inadequate programs, and poor design are the top challenges faced by SCUs. Such challenges require a commitment by administration to resources and policies which support the SCU.

LEARNING EXERCISES

1. If you were locked in a unit all day, every day, what would make it a more pleasant environment for you? List at least five inexpensive changes that would improve the environment.
2. If you could design the perfect SCU, how would it look? How many beds would it have? Where would it be located in your facility? What safety features would it have? What kind of furniture? What type of flooring? What activities?
3. Go on a scavenger hunt around your facility. Find at least 10 activities that demented residents find enjoyable.
4. List at least five helpful hints that every caregiver of a demented person should know about dementia.
5. Plan a nice outdoor wandering area for dementia residents. Where would it be located? What safety features would it have to protect the residents? What kind of benches and gardens would it have?
6. Interview a staff person who works on an SCU. Find out what the benefits and challenges are of taking care of demented residents on an SCU.

POSTTEST

Place a "T" before true statements, an "F" before false statements, and a question mark before those you don't know.

_____ 1. There is consumer demand for SCUs.

_____ 2. SCU residents need the most assistance with eating and toileting.

_____ 3. Residents with a psychiatric diagnosis should be admitted to SCUs.

_____ 4. Staff who work on units other than the SCU should also be trained in dementia.

_____ 5. It is helpful if all facility staff can float onto the SCU.

_____ 6. Good activities for demented residents are dancing and listening to music.

_____ 7. Pets should not be taken onto an SCU as the residents might harm them.

_____ 8. Residents experience agitation when they are bored.

_____ 9. Following training, staff need to be reminded to use their new skills.

_____ 10. A ratio of one staff person to 10 residents has been recommended by the Office of Technology Assessment.

REFERENCES

Buettner, L. (1998). Activities as an intervention for disturbed behavior on the special care unit. In M. Kaplan & S. B. Hoffman (Eds.), *Behaviors in dementia: Best practices for effective management.* Baltimore, MD: Health Professions Press.

Cohen-Mansfield, J., Marx, M. S., & Werner, P. (1992). Observational data on time use and behavior problems in the nursing home. *Journal of Applied Gerontology, 11*(1), 111–121.

Gerdner, L. A., & Buckwalter, K. C. (1996, March/April). Review of state policies regarding Special Care Units: Implications for family consumers and health care professionals. *American Journal of Alzheimer's Disease,* pp. 16–27.

Hoffman, S. B., & Kaplan, M. (1998). Problems encountered in the implementation of special care programs. *American Journal of Alzheimer's Disease, 13,* 197–202.

Kaplan, M. (1996). Special care programs: Challenges to success. In S. B. Hoffman and M. Kaplan (Eds.), *Special care programs for people with dementia* (pp. 1–15). Baltimore, MD: Health Professions Press.

Maas, M. L., Specht, J. P., Weiler, K., Buckwalter, K. C., & Turner, B. (1998). Special care units for people with Alzheimer's Disease: Only for the privileged few? *Journal of Gerontological Nursing, 24*(3), 28–37.

Office of Technology Assessment. (1987). *Losing a million minds: Confronting the tragedy of Alzheimer's disease and other dementias.* Washington, DC: U.S. Congress.

Phillips, C. D., Sloane, P. D., Hawes, C., Koch, G., Han, J., Spry, K., Dunterman, G., & Williams, R. L. (1997). Effects of residence in Alzheimer

---

Answers: 1-T, 2-T, 3-F, 4-T, 5-F, 6-T, 7-F, 8-T, 9-T, 10-F.

Disease special care units on functional outcomes. *Journal of the American Medical Association, 278,* 1340–1344.

Stevens, A., Burgio, L. D., Bailey, E., Burgio, K., Paul, P., Capilouto, E., Nicovich, P., & Hale, G. (1998). Teaching and maintaining behavior management skills with nursing assistants in a nursing home. *Gerontologist, 38,* 379–384.

Chapter **13**

Dying and Grieving

LEARNING OBJECTIVES

- To describe "anticipatory grief"
- To identify three different advanced directives
- To list the important aspects of care for the dying resident
- To identify two ways of helping family members with grieving
- To acknowledge one's own reaction to the deaths of residents

PRETEST

Place a "T" before true statements, an "F" before false statements, and a question mark before those you don't know.

_____ 1. In Alzheimer's disease, the mind and body deteriorate at the same rate until death occurs.

_____ 2. Family members may begin to grieve the loss of a loved one as soon as they learn the loved one is terminally ill.

_____ 3. One should be over grieving the death of a loved one in one year's time.

_____ 4. DNR stands for do not resuscitate.

_____ 5. One problem with getting hospice care for persons with dementia is they are unable to give informed consent for this type of care.

_____ 6. Living Wills are legally recognized and followed in all states.

_____ 7. Palliative care requires aggressively treating all infections with antibiotics.

_____ 8. Because of their dementia, a "good death" is irrelevant to Alzheimer's sufferers.

_____ 9. It is very unlikely that a caregiver in a nursing home would feel bereaved when a resident had died.

_____ 10. Most dementia patients die of infection.

One of the more difficult aspects of nursing home care is the belief on the part of many of the residents and their family members that the resident has been sent there to die. This is a very negative way of looking at nursing home admission. It is true that a great many people who enter a nursing home spend their last days there. But this can be turned into a positive experience if staff, family, and resident are prepared to approach it in a positive way and strive for "a good death."

DEMENTIA AND DYING

Alzheimer's disease and related dementias are terminal illnesses. Their eventual outcome is death. Persons with dementia are at higher risk of dying for several reasons. Throughout the course of the disease, they are at higher risk of accidental death because of the poor judgment that is part of cognitive impairment As the disease progresses, they begin to lose their ability to walk and other motor functions (Brechling, Heyworth, Kuhn, & Peranteau, 1989). This leads to problems associated with decreased mobility including skin breakdown, constipation, and impaired respiratory function. Also, they begin to experience difficulty swallowing. This can lead to the serious problem of aspiration pneumonia.

Despite this progressive decline in ability to function, persons with dementia do not die of dementia per se. Instead they die of some condition that is the result of their poor functional status. Usually they die of an infection. Most dementia victims ultimately die of

Answers: 1-F, 2-T, 3-F, 4-T, 5-T, 6-F, 7-F, 8-F, 9-F, 10-T.

pneumonia (Volicer, Volicer, & Hurley, 1993), but the dementia is the underlying cause.

However, dying from dementia is different from other terminal illnesses in several ways. One difference is the time it takes, up to 10 years or more of progressive decline (Austrum & Hendrie, 1990). Another difference is that the individual with Alzheimer's dementia often remains physically healthy well into the course of the disease, while the mind becomes less and less able to function. The person has a psychological death, or a death of the personality, sometimes years before the actual physical death (Austrum & Hendrie, 1990; Curl, 1992).

ANTICIPATORY GRIEF

Grief is an emotional reaction to loss. When one is aware of the eventuality of a profound loss, such as when there has been a diagnosis of a terminal illness, one often experiences grief in anticipation of the loss. Anticipatory grief is a condition in which a person experiences feelings of grief before an expected loss (Curl, 1992; Fulton, 1987).

Persons who have a terminal illness, and those who love them, often experience anticipatory grief (Fulton, 1987). The person who is dying mourns his or her own death—grieves leaving behind loved ones and giving up goals and dreams for the future. The family and loved ones mourn the coming death of the terminally ill person, the loss of the relationship, and the changes they will need to make in their lives (Walker, Pomeroy, McNeil, & Franklin, 1994).

In the early stages of the disease, while the cognitive impairment is mild, the person who has been diagnosed with Alzheimer's disease may experience anticipatory grieving. As the disease progresses, the increasing cognitive impairment takes away the person's self-awareness and knowledge of what the future holds in store. The family, however, is faced with the continued mental deterioration of their loved one. Eventually, though physically the person with dementia may be fairly healthy and look much the same as he or she always did, he or she is lost to the family because the personality they know is gone. The family may mourn the loss of the personality as if the person had died. At times, this anticipatory grieving can lead to a withdrawal from the person with dementia, a seemingly increasing indifference to them.

When persons with dementia are in a long-term-care facility, they are usually being cared for by staff who only know them as demented persons. The caregivers may find it hard to understand the family's withdrawal.

STAGES OF GRIEF

It has been observed that people tend to respond to a death or other loss with a series of similar emotions. These emotions may be experienced in a different order or in different intensities. However, there are recognizable responses or stages in most people's reaction to a loss. Kubler-Ross (1969) was one of the first to identify the stages of grieving, and her ideas provide a useful framework for discussing these reactions. Kubler-Ross, as well as other writers in this area, emphasize that the stages are not necessarily experienced in any particular order. Also one can go back and forth between stages, reexperiencing an earlier stage after one thought it was resolved and one had moved on (Curl, 1992; Saxon & Etten, 1994).

The stages are described as follows:

• Denial—This may be experienced as shock or numbness and may be the first response to the news of a terminal diagnosis or a death. People may act as if they have not heard the news and go on as if nothing has changed. Denial serves to protect one's emotional well-being, and is beneficial in helping one emotionally survive bad news. But if denial continues for an extended period, one cannot make practical plans or realistic decisions about the future.

• Anger—Anger is a natural response to threat, and the loss of a loved one is a threat to one's well-being. When someone experiences anger during grieving, the target of the anger may be difficult to predict. At times, the target may be the person with the terminal illness or the person who has died. The family member may be furious with this person because he or she got sick or is "leaving/left." At times, the target of the anger may be a physician who gave the bad news or a caregiver. The family member may become excessively critical of the direct care staff and make unjustified complaints. If the caregiver can recognize that this anger is a stage in the grieving process the person is going through, it is easier to be objective and not take the attacks personally.

• Bargaining—At this stage, the person has a realization that the loss is inevitable, but tries to control the circumstances of the loss. The person may seek out different doctors or try new, often unproven, treatments in an effort to delay the inevitable. The person may try to "make deals" with fate such as "Let Mother live until her grandchild is born." These efforts are understandable, but can be frustrating to watch. This is especially true when the efforts seem futile and when financial, emotional, and physical resources that perhaps could be put to better use elsewhere are being used up on treatments of little benefit.

• Depression—When people realize the loss is inevitable and there is nothing they can do to change it, they may experience depression. They may have feelings of hopelessness and helplessness. They may be sad and weepy. They may withdraw and not talk with anyone or have difficulty motivating themselves to do anything because they feel there's no use. When family members are in this stage, they may stop visiting their relative because it's "too upsetting." This is a very painful stage. Persons may also feel shame and guilt during this stage.

• Acceptance—During this stage, people have come to terms with the loss. They know the loss is inevitable, but they accept it. They can go on with day-to-day life, enjoying it for what it is and not being totally focused on and consumed by the loss. At this stage, they are experiencing emotional calm and peace. It tends to be a quiet time and the person may not want to interact with a lot of people.

As mentioned previously, these stages are emotional reactions people typically experience in response to loss or the threat of loss. Thus, they may occur during "anticipatory grief" as well as after a person dies. Some research has shown that the anticipatory grief the family of dementia residents experiences is beneficial. It lessens the grief reaction the family experiences when the demented resident actually dies. Other research did not find this to be so. Anticipatory grieving did not change the grief reaction after the loved one had actually died (Fulton, 1987; Ryan, 1992).

A consequence of successfully reaching acceptance during a period of anticipatory grief is that with reaching acceptance of the loss, the family member may go on with grief work. They may withdraw from the dying person and begin to make a new life for themselves. Because the loved one is still alive, although perhaps too demented to recognize anyone, this behavior by family members may seem inappropriate to others (Cohen & Eisdorfer, 1986; Fulton, 1987).

Walker and her associates (1994) make the point that different family members may be at different stages in their anticipatory grieving. Because of this they may be in conflict among themselves over what is best for the dying resident. This conflict may complicate care of the resident as important decisions may not be made in a timely manner, or decisions thought to have been made may be changed unexpectedly.

ISSUES IN THE CARE OF THE DYING RESIDENT

One of the consequences of the advances in medical science is that questions arise as to how aggressively to treat someone with a terminal illness. In many cases, people can be kept alive long beyond the time when they would have died before there were such medical advances as antibiotics, feeding tubes, respirators, etc. When people are demented and cannot give informed consent for the type/amount of treatment they want, it may be decided that everything should be done to extend their lives. The most aggressive treatments may be instituted. However, with a terminally ill person whose condition is deteriorating, the pain and expense of such treatments may seem excessive and futile. In the end, they may add little time to the person's life. Comfort rather than prolonged survival may be preferred (Collins & Ogle, 1994). Advanced directives are one way to help caregivers make decisions about the types and amount of aggressive treatment a person should receive. However, advanced directives need to be made when a person can understand the consequences of the directive. The person needs to be competent to make such a decision about his or her future.

ADVANCED DIRECTIVES

An advanced directive allows a person to indicate in writing what they wish to be done or not done, should death be near and there is no realistic hope of recovery (Saxon & Etten, 1994). Advanced directives include:

• Living Will—This is a document in which a competent person provides specific instructions about health care treatment they do and do not want, should he or she become terminally ill and unable to make his or her own health care decisions (Saxon & Etten, 1994). The Living Will needs to be specific about life-prolonging procedures such as CPR, antibiotic treatment, IVs, and so on, that are or are not wanted. The Living Will must also specify the circumstances under which such procedures should be used or not used. The document must be signed and witnessed. Although many states consider a Living Will to be a legal document, some states do not. One must be aware of the laws regarding Living Wills and other advanced directives in one's own state.

• Health Care Proxy—This document designates a person to act as a health care agent to make treatment decisions in another person's behalf. Usually, a person designates a family member or trusted friend to act as his or her health care agent should he or she become incapable of making such decisions themselves. The designated health care agent interprets the individual's wishes regarding health care decisions depending on the specific medical circumstances. A Living Will can guide the health care agent in making such decisions. Two witnesses other than the designated health care agent must sign the document. The person designating the health care agent must also sign the document. Health Care Proxies are recognized in all states.

• Durable Power of Attorney—A competent person can appoint another person to act as a durable power of attorney. The appointed person is allowed to make certain financial, legal, or other decisions, including health care decisions, for a specific period of time and under specific circumstances. State laws vary as to who can serve as a durable power of attorney and what powers they can have (Saxon & Etten, 1994).

• Guardian—A guardian is an individual appointed by the court to make decisions regarding property and/or health care matters for a person who has been legally declared incompetent.

• Do-Not-Resuscitate (DNR) Order—This is probably the most common and most specific of the advanced directives. It is a document and doctor's order that tells medical professionals not to perform cardiopulmonary resuscitation (CPR) should the person suffer cardiac arrest. A DNR order for a nursing home resident informs the staff and the emergency medical personnel not to perform emergency resuscitation and not to send the resident to the hospital for such treatment. The order is specific to CPR and does not relate to any other treatment or other decisions about health care outlined in, for instance, a Living Will.

Many nursing home residents with dementia will have DNR orders. It has been found that there is a very low success rate for resuscitation for persons with brain impairment. Even if they are successfully revived, they subsequently experience a faster progression of their dementia (Applebaum, Ring, & Finucane, 1990). Thus, CPR may be counterproductive in residents with mid- or late-stage dementia (Volicer et al., 1993).

Persons who are involved in the day-to-day care of residents with dementia or other terminal illnesses cannot help but have feelings about decisions made either to initiate life-prolonging treatment or to withhold such treatment. Some staff members will strongly believe that life should be supported as long as there is medical knowledge and equipment to prolong it. Others will believe it is inhumane and wasteful of resources to put a terminally ill person through intrusive and painful procedures that may only prolong their lives a few days or weeks. The existence of advanced directives the resident made as a competent person helps staff and family accept decisions with which they might not otherwise agree because the resident's own wishes are clear. It is also important for staff to meet and discuss their feelings about possibly controversial decisions regarding the care of a resident. At such meetings, the rationale for the treatment decision, including the resident's wishes as known through advanced directives and the family's wishes, may be discussed. Ideally, if a staff member finds the care plan for a terminally ill resident unacceptable or impossible to carry out because of religious or philosophical beliefs, that staff member should be allowed to withdraw from the care of that resident. The usual practice, however, is that the staff member who objects will continue to provide routine care but will be excused from administering the particular therapies he or she finds objectionable (Ouslander, Osterweil, & Morley, 1997).

HOSPICE CARE FOR RESIDENTS WITH DEMENTIA

Hospice is a concept of care that provides supportive and palliative care for dying patients and their families. It includes psychological, social, and spiritual dimensions of care as well as physical care (Wilson, Kovach, & Stearns, 1996). It has developed as an alternative way of caring for persons who are terminally ill with cancer when they are thought to have no more than 6 months to live. The hospice-care concept was prompted by the belief that a terminally ill person should have the opportunity to die with "dignity." When there is no longer hope for a cure or a meaningful extension to life, the person should be allowed to have a good death. He or she should be made as comfortable as possible, in pleasant surroundings, in the company of people he or she wants. There is an emphasis on symptom control as well as preparation for death and support of the family and caregivers before and after death (Brechling et al., 1989). In 1983 the federal government extended Medicare and Medicaid to cover hospice care expenses under certain conditions. These conditions include that the person is competent to give informed consent and to make decisions about his or her medical treatment and that the person has an expected life span of 6 months or less.

It is difficult to enroll persons with dementia in formal hospice programs because it is difficult to meet these criteria. Persons with dementia are unable to make decisions for themselves, and it is difficult to predict the duration of survival (Volicer et al., 1993). However, some facilities have made efforts to embrace the hospice concept for their advanced stage dementia residents. The facility may invite hospice workers to work with the resident and family within the nursing home as they would in a private home (Amar, 1994). Alternatively, the facility may set up hospice-style care units or areas within the facility for advanced dementia residents (Wilson et al., 1996). In such circumstances, the focus of care becomes ensuring comfort rather than keeping the resident alive at all costs (Volicer et al., 1993).

The dementia residents in a nursing home hospice care unit are different from traditional hospice patients in several ways (Wilson et al., 1996). The dementia residents have a longer life expectancy, the course of their illness is not predictable, they do not require large doses of narcotics for pain, and they have severe impairment of cognitive and social skills.

The hospice-style program described by Wilson, Kovach, and Stearns (1996) focused on five areas of care—comfort, quality of life, dignity, support of family, and support of staff. These five areas would

seem to be universally important in any program caring for the terminally ill.

COMFORT

Most residents with advanced dementia are unable to verbally communicate their needs. Therefore, it is critically important that nursing
staff be able to evaluate a resident's demeanor and behavior to know
whether the person is experiencing discomfort. One of the signs of
discomfort in a nonverbal resident is persistent agitation. Common
causes of discomfort include constipation and fecal impaction, urinary
tract and other infections, pain from contractures, or arthritic changes.

Wilson and her associates recommend that an individualized comfort care plan be developed for each resident in the hospice-style
program. This plan would include interventions that could be implemented to relieve discomfort. The plan would be individualized by
including interventions that have worked with the resident before.
Some possible interventions include:

• Repositioning to improve comfort
• Massage
• Sensory stimulation through music or through materials to touch
  and manipulate
• Pictures of family members
• Individual attention, one-to-one interaction

As mentioned, one of the possible causes for discomfort in a termi-
nal-stage dementia resident may be infection. There is some controversy about the use of antibiotics to aggressively treat infections in
persons with advanced dementia. Administering antibiotics through
IVs or injections is invasive and potentially painful. The side effects
of powerful antibiotics are often unpleasant (e.g., severe diarrhea).
Also, it has been found that in persons with advanced dementia, infections often quickly return after the antibiotic treatment has been completed (Volicer et al., 1993). Many persons, as part of a Living Will or
Health Care Proxy, indicate that they do not want aggressive antibiotic
treatment for infections when they are terminally ill with dementia.
This is a recognition that infection usually is the cause of death in

dementia. Infections can be treated palliatively to relieve discomfort without the use of powerful antibiotics (Schmitz, Lynn, & Cobbs, 1997).

QUALITY OF LIFE

Quality of life for persons with advanced dementia involves being in pleasant surroundings with daily activities that give one pleasure. The environment should provide the optimal amount of stimulation. Efforts should be made to decrease excessive noise and commotion. Many persons with advanced dementia are unable to respond to or participate in group activities but do respond to individual attention. Caregivers may need educational programs to help them develop meaningful and pleasurable activities for individuals with advanced dementia.

One quality-of-life issue that often develops at the advanced stages of dementia is whether or not to institute tube feeding. As discussed earlier, because swallowing is often a problem and aspiration pneumonia a frequent risk, many residents with advanced dementia are tube fed. A nasal-gastric tube is quite unpleasant to insert and maintain. A gastric tube, which goes directly into the stomach through the abdomen, may be less bothersome to a resident but requires surgery to install and presents the risk of infection at the stoma sight. Often, residents attempt to pull out either such tube. This may require that they be mechanically restrained to prevent them from injuring themselves. Also, they lose the sensory experiences and pleasures of food in the mouth and the taste of food during eating.

Miss Langtry, age 86, had severe COPD. She also had severe dementia. After several hospitalizations for aspiration pneumonia, a gastric peg-tube was inserted in her stomach before she was returned to the long-term-care facility. Miss Langtry was confined to her bed in her room for recovery. She kept trying to pull out the tube so wrist restraints were applied to prevent her from doing this. One time she did remove the tube and it required rehospitalization and more surgery to reinsert it. Miss Langtry gradually recovered to the point where she could sit unrestrained in a Geri-chair in the Common Room. She continued to require wrist restraints while in bed to prevent her from injuring herself by pulling out the tube.

A very controversial situation may occur when a person with advanced dementia is unable to eat or simply stops eating. Some residents may have requested in advanced directives that they not be kept alive by artificial means including tube feedings. Yet, caregivers find the idea of a person in their care essentially starving to death horrific. It has been observed (e.g., Schmitz et al., 1997) that a person who has stopped eating or drinking at the end of life appears calm and at peace. Attempts to force them to be nourished or hydrated through tube feedings or IVs only seems to cause them discomfort and pain and does not significantly add to their lifetime.

HUMAN DIGNITY

One of the most important aspects of hospice-type care, as with all care, is to treat the resident with advanced dementia in a respectful, caring manner. For people with advanced dementia, who cannot provide for any of their own needs, this often means ensuring they maintain a good appearance. They should be clean and free of odor at all times. It also means providing the residents with periods of human interaction at times other than when necessary care is being given. It means trying to perform care in a manner you know from previous experience or family report that they prefer. It means providing diversions and activities (types of music, presence of animals, access to outdoors) that they are known to have enjoyed in the past.

SUPPORT FOR FAMILY

An important part of the hospice concept is providing support for family members as they deal with the terminal illness of their loved one. In applying hospice-type care to persons with advanced dementia, the family needs to be involved and their needs and wishes considered at every step of the way. The family members need to feel comfortable and supported in spending time with their terminally ill loved one. They need this time to help them accept the approaching death and to tie up any "loose ends" that may exist in the relationship. Questioning the family at regular intervals regarding their thoughts and ideas about the care of their loved one is one way of supporting the family. Providing special informational meetings, bulletin boards, or holiday parties for family members will help the families feel more comfortable and familiar with the facility and staff. It will also help staff become more comfortable with residents' families.

SUPPORT FOR STAFF

Caring for persons with terminal illness can be very stressful, especially when the added stress of caring for persons with dementia is considered. Staff members who are to work in a specialized program, such as a hospice-type unit within a long-term-care facility, need to feel supported by the administration. Such support can come by way of the administration sponsoring specialized education for staff in the new program. Administration can also ensure that the program will be properly staffed with trained and experienced caregivers at all times. Staff members within the program should be encouraged to give support to each other. They should be encouraged to share with each other their feelings and experiences in the program. A work atmosphere that supports sharing experiences and feelings can greatly enhance a staff member's comfort and satisfaction with the job.

WHEN THE RESIDENT HAS DIED

Family

It is appropriate for the staff members who have cared for a resident who has died to provide comfort and reassurance to the family. The survivors need to accomplish certain "tasks of mourning" to help them come to terms with their loss and get on with their lives. These tasks, as listed by Schmitz and her associates (1994), are:

1. Accepting the reality of the loss
2. Experiencing the pain of the loss
3. Adjusting to an environment in which the deceased is missing
4. Withdrawing emotional energy from the deceased and reinvesting it in other relationships and activities.

You can help family members begin to accomplish these tasks in several ways. Family members should be called to the bedside of a dying loved one whenever possible. They should be allowed to spend some private time with the body of their loved one after death has occurred. This allows the family members time to adjust to the reality of the death and to say their "good-bye's" to their loved one.

The family should be encouraged to talk about the deceased and to be listened to when they want to express their grief. Staff members can share their own positive memories of the resident with family members. Staff members can also suggest appropriate community resources that might be helpful to the family.

Staff Members

People who work in long-term care provide extensive and intimate care for a resident, sometimes for years. It is natural for the staff member to experience some feelings when the resident dies. The resident is an individual who has been a part of your life and when he or she dies, you experience a loss.

It is important that you acknowledge to yourself that you do feel a loss and deal with the feelings in an appropriate way. Staff "burnout" is common in situations where residents frequently die. Burnout is exacerbated when staff do not acknowledge that they experience feelings of loss and grief when residents in their care die.

One way of acknowledging feelings of loss and grief is to have a working environment that accepts feelings and encourages staff members to talk among themselves about their feelings and sense of loss when a resident dies. It is important to allow the acknowledgment of negative feelings about the resident who has been unpleasant and difficult to care for. Verbalizing such feelings in a supportive and understanding atmosphere of fellow workers can help relieve feelings of guilt over "thinking ill of the dead." Such discussions can help you see the positive aspects of the resident and of your job.

Attending a memorial service is another way of addressing your feelings about the death of a resident. If you have been particularly close to the resident or family, you may wish to attend the resident's funeral. Some long-term-care facilities regularly schedule services or other gatherings where they memorialize residents who have died. Such services can be healing experiences for staff and residents alike. These gatherings should be handled in a way that avoids dwelling on the number of deaths and the pain of the dying. They should instead celebrate the lives of the deceased and the good deaths they achieved.

SUMMARY

This chapter is concerned with issues surrounding dying and the death of residents with advanced dementia. It discusses the anticipatory grief the resident and his or her family may experience when they learn the resident is terminally ill. It describes advanced directives residents may have established, which can guide the extent and scope of health care interventions when the resident is no longer capable of expressing his or her wishes. The implementation of hospice-type care for residents who are in the last stages of dementia is also described. It is noted that family members need to be involved in the dying process of their loved one and also need to be supported by long-term-care staff after their loved one has died. Finally, the need for staff to recognize their own feelings of loss when a resident in their care has died is addressed.

LEARNING EXERCISES

1. Think of a resident in your care who has died. Describe your feelings about the death and what happened afterwards. State what you think went well and what you would like to have changed.
2. Have you established advanced directives for yourself? Who would you appoint as a health care agent or to whom would you give durable power of attorney? Does that person know your wishes regarding life-prolonging procedures should you be unable to make such decisions yourself? Briefly outline a Living Will expressing your preferences for health care procedures should you have a terminal illness.
3. Describe the components of a hospice-type care program you would design for persons with advanced dementia. What special education would you provide for staff working in the program? What activities would you provide for residents of the program? How would you involve family members? What other features would you have in your program?

4. Discuss your feelings about caring for terminally ill residents. What is your idea of a "good death" for a person with advanced dementia? How do you feel about withholding medical procedures such as antibiotic therapy, tube feedings, IV hydration, or respirators for persons in the terminal stage of dementia?

POSTTEST

Place a "T" before true statements, an "F" before false statements, and a question mark before those you don't know.

     1. Family members who have experienced "anticipatory grief" may start to withdraw from their terminally ill loved one before the person has actually died.

     2. Persons with Alzheimer's disease rarely die of pneumonia.

     3. A Health Care Proxy designates a person to make health care decisions for someone who is incompetent to make such decisions for himself or herself.

     4. It is very unusual for a grieving person to feel angry.

     5. It's useless to complete advanced directives because no one follows them anyway.

     6. Hospice care concepts can be applied to persons who are in the advanced stages of dementia.

     7. Staff members caring for terminally ill dementia residents benefit from sharing their experiences and feelings with each other.

     8. It is harmful to allow family members to spend time with the body of their resident who has died.

     9. Everyone experiences stages of grieving in the same order and in the same way.

     10. Hospice care promotes making the dying person as comfortable as possible, in pleasant surroundings, in the company of his or her loved ones.

Answers: I-T, 2-F, 3-T, 4-F, 5-F, 6-T, 7-T, 8-F, 9-F, 10-T.

REFERENCES

Amar, D. F. (1994). The role of the hospice social worker in the nursing home setting. *American Journal of Hospice and Palliative Care, 11,* 18–23.

Applebaum, G. E., Ring, J. E., & Finucane, T. E. (1990). The outcome of CPR initiated in nursing homes. *Journal of the American Geriatrics Society, 38,* 197–200.

Austrom, M. G., & Hendrie, H. C. (1990). Death of the personality: The grief response of the Alzheimer's disease family caregiver. *American Journal of Alzheimer's Care and Related Disorders and Research, 5,* 16–27.

Brechling, B. G., Hayworth, J. A., Kuhn, D., & Peranteau, M. F. (1989). Extending hospice care to end-stage dementia patients and families. *American Journal of Alzheimer's Care and Related Disorders and Research, 4,* 21–29.

Cohen, D., & Eisdorfer, C. (1986). *The loss of self.* New York: Norton.

Collins, C., & Ogle, K. (1994). Patterns of predeath service use by dementia patients with a family caregiver. *Journal of the American Geriatrics Society, 42,* 719–722.

Curl, A. (1992, Nov./Dec.). When family caregivers grieve for the Alzheimer's patient. *Geriatric Nursing,* pp. 305–307.

Fulton, R. (1987). The many faces of grief. *Death Studies, 11,* 243–256.

Kubler-Ross, E. (1969). *On death and dying.* New York: Macmillan.

Ouslander, J. G., Osterweil, D., & Morley, J. (1997). Hospice care and pain management. In *Medical care in the nursing home* (2nd ed., pp. 419–429). New York: McGraw-Hill.

Ryan, D. H. (1992). Is there a desolation effect after dementia? A comparative study of mortality rates in spouses of dementia patients following admission and bereavement. *International Journal of Geriatric Psychiatry, 7,* 331–339.

Saxon, S. V., & Etten, M. J. (1994). Death and grief in the later years. In *Physical change and aging* (pp. 376–405). New York: Tiresias Press.

Schmitz, P., Lynn, J., & Cobbs, E. (1994). The care of the dying patient. In W. R. Hazzard, E. Bierman, J. P. Blass, W. H. Ettinger, & J. B. Halter (Eds)., *Principles of geriatric medicine and gerontology* (3rd ed., pp. 383–390). New York: McGraw-Hill.

Volicer, L., Volicer, B. J., & Hurley, A. C. (1993). Is hospice care appropriate for Alzheimer's patients? *Caring, 12,* 50–55.

Walker, R. J., Pomeroy, E. C., McNeil, J. S., & Franklin, C. (1994). Anticipatory grief and Alzheimer's disease: Strategies for intervention. *Journal of Gerontological Social Work, 22,* 21–39.

Wilson, S. A., Kovach, C. R., & Stearns, S. A. (1996). Hospice concepts in the care of end-stage dementia. *Geriatric Nursing, 17,* 6–10.

Index